OSPITAL

RY - Ext 6227

SLEEP DISORDERS

CURRENT ◊ CLINICAL ◊ PRACTICE

SLEEP DISORDERS

DIAGNOSIS AND TREATMENT

Edited by

J. STEVEN POCETA, MD

and

MERRILL M. MITLER, PhD

*Scripps Clinic and
The Scripps Institute, La Jolla, CA*

Foreword by

SHIRLEY OTIS, MD

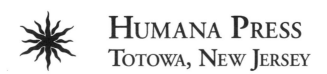

HUMANA PRESS
TOTOWA, NEW JERSEY

© 1998 Humana Press Inc.
999 Riverview Drive, Suite 208
Totowa, New Jersey 07512

For additional copies, pricing for bulk purchases, and/or information about other Humana titles,
contact Humana at the above address or at any of the following numbers: Tel: 973-256-1699;
Fax: 973-256-8341; E-mail: humana@humanapr.com

Cover design by Patricia F. Cleary

This publication is printed on acid-free paper.∞
ANSI Z39.48-1984 (American National Standards Institute) Permanence of Paper for Printed
Library Materials).

Printed in the United States of America. 10 9 8 7 6 5 4 3 2 1

FOREWORD

Everyone sleeps! Sleep is that familiar to us all, yet still remains a medical mystery. The Britannica definition "*the normal periodic suspension of consciousness during which the powers of the body are restored*" takes into account the essential nature of sleep for optimal human well-being. This has been known since time immemorial. The fear and problems of inadequate sleep are expressed in a quote from Henry IV:

> O Sleep, O gentle Sleep!
> Nature's soft nurse, how have I
> frightened thee,
> That thou no more wilt weigh mine eyelids down
> and steep my senses in forgetfulness?
>
> *Shakespeare*: Henry IV III.i.

Despite many remarkable advances in the study of disorders of sleep, including a new appreciation of the physiologic, endocrinologic, and biologic processes involved, this knowledge has not been well-disseminated to the public nor to the physicians caring for them. Thus, although our knowledge base has increased exponentially, sleep disorders remain a significant and under-treated public health problem.

At a time when cost consciousness is pervasive in medicine, the total costs to the public resulting from sleep disorders is almost impossible to estimate. The costs include the risks from the association of sleep apnea with stroke, headache, and hypertension, as well as the costs associated with accidents because of sleep deprivation. Even with the wealth of information regarding sleep disorders available to us, their importance and treatment have not been emphasized in our medical training or clinical practices. Most of the knowledge of the diagnosis and treatment of sleep disorders has existed in small laboratory and specialty-based centers. Many victims of sleep disorders go unaided because of this ignorance.

As American medicine has trended toward the primary care physician as director of medical care (versus specialist-directed care), it becomes increasingly important for our primary care physicians to be knowledgeable about disorders of sleep. Nowhere has the trend toward primary-driven health care been more revolutionary than here at the Scripps Clinic. Over the last six years, Scripps has transitioned from a primarily multispecialty clinic to a greater than 50% primary care physician facility. This trend may be welcomed by some and scorned by others, but for conditions as common as insomnia and snoring, no physician is better positioned for intervention than the primary care physician. Here at Scripps Clinic, we have emphasized the cooperation of specialist and generalist in those areas where the greatest impact can be made.

We therefore welcome this informative, clear, and concise book aimed at the education of primary care providers for improvement in patient care delivery. The authors of these chapters have been carefully selected to present current expert opinion in a reader-friendly way, emphasizing a practical approach to the disorders. The primary care physician will find that these chapters elucidate sleep complaints and their relationship to common clinical syndromes. The book is clearly and logically organized, easily readable, and should stand as an authoritative work for primary physicians for many years to come.

Shirley Otis, MD

PREFACE

The field of sleep disorders medicine has expanded rapidly in the United States and around the world. Before the 1970s, the study of sleep was an area populated by a few neurologists, psychiatrists, and physiologists. With the recognition that obstructive sleep apnea is a common clinical condition and that many common drugs produce undesirable sedation during the day, the field has grown rapidly. Individual membership in the American Sleep Disorders Association has increased from fewer than 400 members in 1984 to more than 2400 members in 1996. Most hospitals and medical groups now have routine access to sleep disorders consultations and laboratories. Physicians in virtually any type of practice will encounter patients with some form of sleep disorder, be it obstructive sleep apnea after extubation, or insomnia in a patient with depression.

Primary care physicians routinely see patients in whom the chief complaint suggests a specific sleep disorder, or in whom a sleep disorder indirectly influences their medical condition. *Sleep Disorders'* major goal is to educate general practitioners in several areas of the clinical practice of sleep disorders medicine. The authors have striven to provide timely and experience-based advice that would be of daily, practical use to any physician. The emphasis is firmly on practice: History-taking, physical examination, differential diagnosis, utilization of laboratory tests, appropriate use of consultation, and treatments. Certain chapters repeat elements found in others—these points are usually important aspects of a common problem, such as determining the cause of insomnia. We hope that after reading *Sleep Disorders: Diagnosis and Treatment*, the reader will have a working knowledge of sleep-related conditions, and thus will be able to approach patients suffering disorders of sleep in full confidence.

Dr. Patrick Strollo is an active clinician and researcher as well as a member of the American Sleep Disorders Association committee on primary care education. He offers a broad perspective on the evaluation of patients with sleep disorders in a general practice, and elaborates on the details of history-taking and physical examination. As in any field, there are a series of questions whose answers are instrumental to the proper assessment of sleep disorder complaints, and many aspects of the sleep disorders history are not appreciated by those outside the field. Thus, the chapter presents a method to develop and expand upon any sleep related complaint, including sleepiness in the day, fatigue, snoring, or insomnia.

Five chapters are devoted to specific conditions that are common in the field of sleep disorders. Dr. Kingman Strohl reviews the many aspects of obstructive sleep apnea. His chapter discusses pathophysiology in sufficient depth for one to understand the typical presentations, symptoms, and therapeutic approach. There is an emphasis on screening procedures, as well as on risk stratification. Dr. J. Steven Poceta, a neurologist and sleep specialist at Scripps Clinic, discusses the restless legs syndrome, which is a condition increasingly recognized by both patients and physicians. A practical approach to diagnosis and treatment is given. Drs. Rafael Pellayo and Christian Guilleminault have world-renowned expertise in the diagnosis and treatment of central nervous system conditions such as narcolepsy. They review diagnostic criteria, typical presentations, "red flags" in the history, as well as treatment options. Dr. Milton Erman, our colleague at the Scripps Clinic, has a busy practice in sleep disorders as well as research interest in insomnia. He has written numerous papers and chapters on insomnia and its treatment, and is active in several trials of behavioral, medical, and other treatments. He approach is both intellectually stimulating and practical. His description of insomnia and his approach to differential diagnosis will remove the frustration and puzzlement that occur in many practitioners facing such patients. Dr. Daniel Kripke is a recognized expert in circadian rhythms, affective disorder, and bright light therapy. He is also a practicing sleep disorders specialist whose chapter on circadian rhythm disturbances and seasonal affective disorder will be useful in assessing patients with almost any sleep or emotional complaint. Practical aspects of the use of bright light therapy are included for the treatment of jet lag.

Drs. Wallace Mendelson and Cosmo Caruso discuss the pharmacology of benzodiazepines, other hypnotic-sedatives, tricyclic antidepressants, serotonin reuptake inhibitors, and stimulants. Dr. Ronald Dahl provides a detailed overview of sleep disorders in children, emphasizing common sleep complaints and common sleep disorders in various age groups. Dr. Stephen Johnson is the Director of the Western Montana Medical Clinic, holds an MBA, and started his clinic's sleep center in 1994. In his chapter, considerations are given to the cost-benefit analysis of diagnosing and treating sleep disorders, as well as the approach to sleep disorders from a managed-care perspective. An emphasis on evolving technologies and protocols should help the reader understand the multitude of factors involved in clinical decision making in this area.

Drs. Richard Simon, Eric Ball, and Jennings Falcon present their experience when the Walla Walla Clinic set out to train a clinician and set up a sleep lab. Their chapter clarifies the fact that patients with sleep disorders are often overlooked in primary care, but that with education and training, recognition of these disorders is beneficial to patients.

We wish to thank all our authors for their fine efforts. It was a pleasure working with such knowledgable and hard-working professionals. We hope that *Sleep Disorders* will be found as helpful to primary care physicians worldwide as we intended.

J. Steven Poceta, MD
Merrill M. Mitler, PhD

CONTENTS

CONTRIBUTORS

ERIC M. BALL, MD, FACP • *Kathryn Severyns Dement Sleep Disorders Center, Department of Medicine, St. Mary Medical Center, Walla Walla Clinic, Walla Walla, WA*

COSMO CARUSO, MD • *Pulmonary Physicians of Kansas City, Inc., Kansas City, MO*

RONALD DAHL, MD • *Child and Adolescent Sleep Laboratory, Departments of Psychiatry and Pediatrics, Western Psychiatric Institute and Clinic, Pittsburgh, PA*

MILTON K. ERMAN, MD • *Department of Psychiatry, University of California, San Diego, CA; The Scripps Research Institute, La Jolla, CA; California Sleep Monitoring, Inc., La Jolla, CA; Division of Neurology, Scripps Clinic, La Jolla, CA*

JENNINGS C. FALCON II, MD • *Kathryn Severyns Dement Sleep Disorders Center, Department of Neurology, St. Mary Medical Center, Walla Walla Clinic, Walla Walla, WA*

CHRISTIAN GUILLEMINAULT, MD • *Sleep Disorder Clinic, Department of Psychiatry, Stanford University Medical Center, Palo Alto, CA*

STEPHEN F. JOHNSON, MD, MBA • *St. Patrick Hospital Sleep Center, Missoula, MT; Western Montana Clinic, Missoula, MT; VRI/Managed Care Montana, Missoula, MT*

DANIEL F. KRIPKE, MD • *Department of Psychiatry, University of California, San Diego, CA*

WALLACE B. MENDELSON, MD • *Sleep Research Laboratory, University of Chicago, Chicago, IL*

RAFAEL PELAYO, MD • *Sleep Disorder Clinic, Department of Psychiatry, Stanford University Medical Center, Palo Alto, CA*

J. STEVEN POCETA, MD • *Division of Neurology, Scripps Clinic, La Jolla, CA; Department of Neuropharmacology, The Scripps Research Institute, La Jolla, CA*

RICHARD D. SIMON, JR., MD • *Kathryn Severyns Dement Sleep Disorders Center, Department of Medicine, St. Mary Medical Center, Walla Walla Clinic, Walla Walla, WA*

KINGMAN P. STROHL, MD • *Center for Sleep Disorders Research, Department of Medicine, Case Western Reserve University and Veterans Affairs Medical Center, Cleveland, OH*

PATRICK J. STROLLO, JR., MD, FCCP, FABSM • *Pulmonary Sleep Disorders Laboratory, Division of Pulmonary, Allergy, and Critical Care Medicine, University of Pittsburgh, Pittsburgh, PA*

1

Sleep Disorders in Primary Care
The History and Physical Examination

Patrick J. Strollo, Jr.

CONTENTS

1. INTRODUCTION

The proper office evaluation of a patient with a sleep disorder requires the ability to establish an appropriate clinical suspicion on the basis of the history and physical examination. Patients frequently suffer in silence owing to two primary factors: most physicians are inadequately trained to inquire about and recognize the variety of sleep disorders that might afflict a patient, and many patients are reluctant to volunteer information regarding the quality and quantity of their sleep because they are either not fully aware of the problem themselves or are uncertain that sleep-related problems are important *(1–3)*. Overlooking sleep-related problems represents a missed opportunity to improve a patient's quality of life and to modify the morbidity and mortality associated with certain specific disorders.

This chapter deals with the fundamental aspects of the sleep history by providing a starting point for the primary care practitioner in identifying common sleep disorders. The focus will be on adults; a separate chapter in this book considers sleep disorders in children. Use of the

From: *Sleep Disorders: Diagnosis and Treatment*
Edited by: J. S. Poceta and M. M. Mitler © Humana Press Inc., Totowa, NJ

term "sleep-disordered breathing" refers to intermittent decrements of ventilation occurring only during sleep. Such respiratory events can be either obstructive in nature (increased upper airway resistance) or can be central (decreased drive to breath). When associated with a clinical syndrome such as restless sleep and daytime sleepiness, the term sleep apnea can be used.

2. THE SLEEP HISTORY

2.1. Normal Sleep

Sleep is a dynamic process which occurs naturally in humans in either one long nocturnal period or in a nocturnal period and an afternoon (siesta) period. Some understanding of normal sleep is helpful in taking a sleep history in order to distinguish the important aspects of the information provided. Some knowledge of normal sleep is assumed, and the interested reader can see ref. 24 for more detail. Sleep is composed of 2 major subtypes—nonREM and REM. NonREM sleep is divided into stages 1, 2, 3, and 4 and is based on the degree of EEG slowing and certain EEG patterns. Stage 1 is "light" sleep, occurring at the transition from wakefulness; stage 2 is the most prevalent stage, and stages 3 and 4 are considered "deep" or "slow-wave" sleep. Stages 3 and 4 occur primarily in the first and second sleep cycle, early in the night.

REM sleep occurs at the end of each sleep cycle (every 90–120 min), and the REM periods last from a few minutes to up to forty minutes, and become longer and more prevalent as the night progresses (see Fig. 1). REM sleep is associated with marked diminution of skeletal muscle tone, the report of dreaming, and autonomic nervous system variability. Knowledge of these basic facts can elucidate pathology—for example, the timing of events such as sleepwalking, insomnia, and headaches.

Physiologic circadian forces cause humans to sleep each night, and these same forces act in a similar manner to produce the "afternoon dip" or siesta. The exact timing of the major sleep period and its phase relationship to the sun seems inherently determined in any individual. Normally, sleep occurs sometime after sunset and ends sometime near dawn. The usual sleep requirement for adults is between seven and nine hours each night. People become excessively sleepy in the day because either the quality or quantity of sleep is disturbed, in combination with the intrinsic circadian rhythm. The issue of daytime sleepiness is of great importance, not only for the individual with the sleep disorder, but in transportation and industrial safety policy-making. A more detailed discussion of sleep and circadian rhythms appears elsewhere in this book.

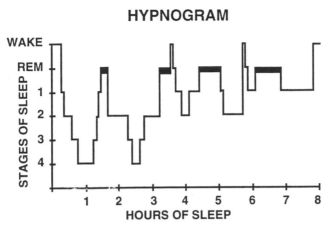

Fig. 1. This idealized hypnogram illustrates the usual progression of sleep stages in the normal young adult. There are several basic features of this dynamic process. Early in the night are one or two cycles in which slow wave sleep occurs (stage 3 or 4) followed by a REM period. The initial time to the first REM (REM latency) is usually 60–100 minutes and is altered in certain conditions such as depression or narcolepsy. With subsequent cycles, the occurrence of slow wave sleep is less, and the duration of REM periods longer. In the elderly, there is less or no slow wave sleep, and generally more disruption (wake time) throughout the night.

2.2. Addressing Sleep Complaints

Insomnia and obstructive sleep-disordered breathing are two conditions that are found commonly in middle-aged and elderly adults and, occasionally, in children. Ten percent of adults are troubled by chronic insomnia, and 2–4% of middle-aged adults have sleep apnea *(4,5)*. Thus, investigating only these two conditions in a general population can be rewarding. In adults, a few simple questions can direct the history and physical in order to identify patients "at risk" for these and other sleep disorders. Inquiring about the following can be extremely revealing:

1. The restorative nature of the patient's sleep.
2. Excessive daytime sleepiness, tiredness, or fatigue.
3. The presence of habitual snoring.
4. Whether the total sleep time is sufficient.

The pneumonic *REST* can help the clinician remember these four key questions in the screening history (Table 1).

If there is some kind of complaint about sleep or sleep quality, or if the physician uncovers an area of concern about sleep that could relate

Table 1
Four Key Questions in Screening History

R estorative sleep?
E xcessive daytime sleepiness, tiredness, or fatigue?
S noring nightly?
T otal sleep time?

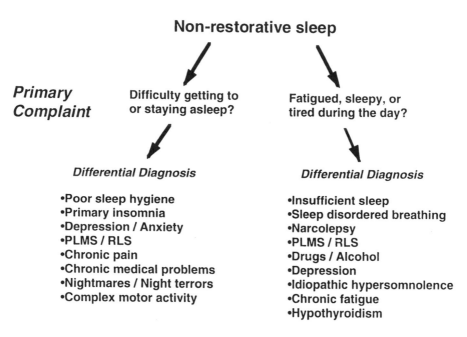

Non-restorative sleep

Primary Complaint

Difficulty getting to or staying asleep?

Fatigued, sleepy, or tired during the day?

Differential Diagnosis

•Poor sleep hygiene
•Primary insomnia
•Depression / Anxiety
•PLMS / RLS
•Chronic pain
•Chronic medical problems
•Nightmares / Night terrors
•Complex motor activity

Differential Diagnosis

•Insufficient sleep
•Sleep disordered breathing
•Narcolepsy
•PLMS / RLS
•Drugs / Alcohol
•Depression
•Idiopathic hypersomnolence
•Chronic fatigue
•Hypothyroidism

Fig. 2. The major diagnostic considerations depending on the complaint are illustrated. It is often useful to characterize the major complaint as being that of either insomnia or daytime sleepiness. In practice, however, certain conditions which present classically with sleepiness such as sleep apnea syndrome occasionally present with insomnia; some cases of depression or conditioned insomnia might occasionally present with fatigue.

to the patient's well-being, the first step in clinical evaluation is to determine if the complaint is primarily about nocturnal sleep or about daytime functioning. Most sleep disorders present as either insomnia or as daytime sleepiness. Insomnia can be of three general types: a complaint of difficulty with initial sleep onset, a complaint of frequent awakenings, or a complaint of waking up too early. Daytime dysfunction can be variably described by the patient as either fatigue, feeling nonrestored by his or her night of sleep, trouble with mental alertness,

Table 2
Sleep History

Bedtime/sleep period
1. Lights out/lights on
2. Time to sleep onset
3. Leg cramps/paraesthesias
4. Pain
Sleep continuity
1. Awakenings—why, how many, how long, activities during
2. Nocturia
3. Nocturnal angina
4. Nocturnal palpitations
5. Nocturnal dyspnea
6. Nocturnal reflux
7. Nocturnal pain, including headache
8. Nightmares/night terrors
9. Complex motor activity
Daytime function
1. Condition upon arising
2. Epworth Sleepiness Scale
3. Driving (accidents)
4. Attention and concentration
5. Cataplexy
Special considerations
1. Bedroom environment
2. Weekends (physiologic jet lag)
3. Shift work
4. Exercise
5. Light exposure
6. Caffeine, tobacco, alcohol ingestion

or frank daytime sleepiness such as falling asleep while driving. Of course, many patients have complaints about both the night and the day; in fact, for insomnia to be considered pathologic, there must be a concomitant complaint not only of nocturnal wakefulness, but also of daytime dysfunction. Nonetheless, most patients can be separated into one of these predominant categories, and this distinction is useful in narrowing the differential diagnosis and directing the work-up (Fig. 2).

A careful sleep history can provide additional information that is frequently overlooked in the standard history. Table 2 breaks down the sleep history into four sections that cover the 24-hour day. One must make specific and directed inquiries about the period immediately before sleep, the night itself, the daytime, and any special aspects of the patient's

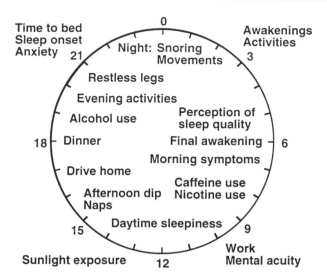

Fig. 3. This diagram illustrates the major components of the 24-hour history. The clock emphasizes that history taking for sleep-wake disorders involves questioning about activities and their timing during the 24-hour day, not just specific symptoms (courtesy of Poceta JS and Mitler MM).

situation. Information about each period might come not only from the patient, but sometimes also from an observer. In general, it is necessary to understand each of these periods in any patient with a sleep complaint. Figure 3 emphasizes the 24-hour nature of the sleep history and its major components.

2.3. Bedtime/Sleep Period

When evaluating a patient with a possible sleep disorder, it is essential to determine the total sleep time that the patient is allowing him or herself to achieve, as well as whether the bedtime and wake-up times are regular or erratic. Most people require eight hours of sleep to feel fully rested. Shorter sleep periods can result in chronic sleep deprivation (sleep restriction or insufficient sleep). Therefore, it is usually necessary to ask the patient what time he or she gets into bed and at what time the lights go out and sleep begins. At the other end of the night, it is necessary to determine at what time the patient awakens and at what time he or she gets out of bed to start the day. A simple way of gaining insight into whether the time allotted for sleep is sufficient for the patient is to ask if an alarm clock is used to awaken each morning and if the patient catches up by sleeping more on weekends and vacations. Insufficient sleep time is the first possibility to eliminate when considering the complaint of sleepiness or fatigue. For many people nowadays, the pre-sleep evening hours is a time to catch up on paperwork or to sign onto a computer service, thus prolonging the bedtime beyond what it might be otherwise. For a patient with the complaint of sleepiness or fatigue, this is often a time when a family member will report that the patient dozes in front of the television; for many patients with sleep-onset insomnia, this is a time the patient begins certain activities or watches television in bed. Also a problem is an erratic sleep schedule with differing bedtimes and wake-up times. The physician must determine the range of variation on workdays vs weekends, for example. Also, the patient's innate circadian tendencies must be evaluated—whether a morning person or a night owl.

Once the physician has a modest understanding of the patient's schedule, one inquires about physical and mental experiences during this period. The pre-sleep period is often the time in which many physical problems are magnified, either because of a true circadian tendency or because the patient is more sedentary and less distracted. Thus, chronic pain from almost any cause can interfere with sleep onset and is often worse in the evening and night. Leg cramps, neuropathic pains, or restless leg syndrome (*see* Chapter 4) can all interfere with sleep onset. In many patients with insomnia, the evening and pre-sleep times are when the "mind is racing" or the patient "can't shut the mind off" and when anxiety and frustration are high. The patient might toss and turn in bed for hours with worry before sleep comes. Whatever the type of complaint and final diagnosis, significant historical clues come from the patient's activities and experiences in the immediate hours before going to sleep.

2.4. Sleep Continuity

Just as sleep onset can be affected by many factors, so, too, can the quality and experience of sleep over the course of the night be negatively impacted by a variety of conditions. Information about sleep quality can further direct the work-up of a suspected sleep disorder. Specifically, one must ask the patient what he or she experiences overnight—if and when do awakenings occur? What seems to cause the awakening? What does the patient do during the awakening? How long does it last? Is there evidence of restlessness (sheets messed up)? Other specifics can be inquired about, depending on the conditions being considered. For example, sometimes dream experiences must be discussed as a clue to whether the problem might be linked to REM sleep. The bedpartner or other observer must also contribute the information that the patient will usually know little about: snoring, movements, and breathing patterns during sleep itself. The pattern of awakenings can suggest specific diagnoses. Conditioned insomnia and anxiety, for example, will typically produce sleep-onset insomnia and not multiple brief arousals in the night—intrinsic sleep-disrupting conditions such as sleep apnea and nocturnal myoclonus are more likely to do that. Patients with obstructive sleep-disordered breathing can also report nocturia, nocturnal angina, nocturnal palpitations, nocturnal diaphoresis, headache upon awakening, or nocturnal dyspnea, in addition to more commonly recognized symptoms such as habitual snoring, nocturnal gasping, snorting, and observed apnea *(6,7)*. Depression typically produces a "terminal insomnia," also called early morning awakening. Pure circadian rhythm disturbances typically produce sound continuous sleep, but which comes too early (thus producing early morning waking) or too late (thus producing sleep-onset insomnia).

However, no strict relationship exists between the pattern of arousals and any specific diagnosis. Obstructive sleep apnea can present as sleep maintenance insomnia. The cause of the arousal might be different than what prolongs the arousal. For example, a dog barking or a leg jerk might awaken a patient, but if the patient is so inclined, beginning to worry about the stress of paying the bills prolongs the arousal. In such a case, it might be better to treat the leg jerks (or silence the dog) than to begin treatment for anxiety.

Nocturia in male patients is almost always interpreted by the physician to be a sign of prostatic hypertrophy. However, in a patient with obstructive sleep apnea (OSA), nocturnal oxyhemoglobin desaturations can trigger hypoxic vasoconstriction that can result in elevated right heart pressures. This rise in right heart pressures stimulates the release of atrial natriuretic peptide (ANP), which results in increased urine formation, thus promoting nocturnal urination *(8)*. Nocturia caused by OSA is typically seen in patients with more severe forms of the disease. Treatment has been shown to decrease the frequency of urination as well as ANP levels.

Patients with OSA may also experience nocturnal angina and palpitations *(9,10)*. Concomitant coronary artery disease or severe OSA is usually found in these patients and should prompt the clinician to refer expediently the patient for definitive evaluation and treatment.

Occasionally, patients with sleep apnea will report nocturnal dyspnea. This can be confused with congestive heart failure caused by ischemic coronary artery disease. Although ischemia can certainly occur (particularly during REM sleep-related desaturations), the sensation of not breathing or of dyspnea can also be a result of arousal without relief of airway occlusion. When OSA is the cause of awakening with a choking or inability to breathe, assuming an upright position and the return of full consciousness promptly relieve the complaint. Paroxysmal nocturnal dyspnea in association with congestive heart failure has a longer temporal profile from the arousals of sleep apnea. Larygospasm from different causes, particularly from gastroesophageal reflux, can produce a complete closure of the (laryngeal) airway, and often, this can continue for many seconds or a minute after awakening. Stridor, and the recognition of inability to move air in or out are clues to this diagnosis. However, nocturnal gastroesophageal reflux can be found in patients with primary acid reflux problems, as well as in patients with sleep apnea. The very negative intrathoracic pressures that are generated in patients with OSA promote reflux by off-setting lower esophageal sphincter tone *(11)*.

Poorly controlled nocturnal pain may also alter sleep continuity. This has been described in patients with arthritis and fibromyalgia/fibromyositis (*see* Chapter 2). In addition, chronic medical problems such as obstructive lung disease, heart disease, or renal disease can impair sleep continuity. Also, medications such as theophylline can interfere with sleep maintenance. In fact, medical causes of insomnia or poor sleep quality should be considered common—but not necessarily untreatable. A variety of strategies are outlined in this volume for dealing with insomnia, even when caused by an untreatable condition such as diabetic peripheral neuropathy.

Sleep paralysis is a interesting symptom that is common in patients with narcolepsy, as well as in individuals that are profoundly REM sleep deprived *(12)*. It is characterized by the inability to move despite being awake, around the time of sleep onset. This represents the direct transition to REM sleep from the waking state. The experience is usually described by the patient as very frightening; it is not uncommon, occurs once or twice in a normal lifetime, and is of no diagnostic significance. When associated with sleepiness or other symptoms or when frequent, sleep paralysis can be a clue to narcolepsy or might need treatment in and of itself. A familial tendency has been reported in the literature on the subject.

Nightmares (frightening dreams occurring during REM sleep) and night terrors ("terrifying" incomplete arousals from deep nonREM sleep without dream recall) can also impact negatively on sleep continuity and sometimes must be inquired about directly. Many patients consider weird dreams to represent some hidden aspect of their mind; thus, they are reluctant to tell others about them for fear of being considered psychologically ill. This is not necessarily untrue—unusual dream experiences can occur as a result of medical illnesses (*see* REM behavior disorder in Chapter 4), as a result of psychologic distress (post traumatic stress disorder or an equivalent), or can be normal. Nightmares and night terrors are most common in children, are usually infrequent, and considered normal. When frequent in children or when persisting into adulthood, nightmares and night terrors can be manifestations of significant neurologic (e.g., seizures) or psychiatric (e.g., abuse) problems. These parasomnias are reviewed in Chapter 8.

Unusual activities or behavior during the sleep period can be manifested by sleeptalking or sleepwalking. The former is relatively common and generally of no consequence, although sleeptalking seems to be more common in those with sleepwalking or REM behavior disorder. Much of what the patient "says" during sleep is unintelligible. Sleepwalking in adults is uncommon. At times, this parasomnia can place the patient in dangerous situations (e.g., if the patient leaves the home or walks unto a balcony). Other complex motor activity can range from nocturnal limb movements, to nocturnal dystonia, to nocturnal seizures, to the REM sleep behavior disorder *(13)*.

Movements of the limbs in the evening and night, called periodic limb movements of sleep (PLMS), can fragment sleep, resulting in poor sleep quality. These sleep-related limb movements can also occur during the waking hours and often are associated with restless leg symptoms. The restless leg syndrome (RLS) manifests as an uncontrollable urge to move the legs and a "crawling" sensation in the legs that can interfere with sleep onset, as well as sleep continuity. Although this condition can occur throughout the night, most patients report their worst restlessness in the evening and early sleep period and their best sleep in the early morning. Often, the patient is unaware of the movements that occur in sleep and is even unaware of the movements that might awaken him or her. The bedpartner can often describe the periodic (every 20–40 s) rhythmic stereotyped movements. Patients with this disorder also typically disrupt the bedcovers are "all over the bed." Some of our patients have presented with the history that they sleep on the floor so that they have more room to move and will not fall out of bed.

The REM sleep behavior disorder deserves special mention. This parasomnia occurs during REM sleep and can be associated with injury to the patient or the bedpartner. It is characterized by a loss of the muscle atonia that normally accompanies REM sleep and can result in the patient "acting out " dream imagery (e.g., being chased or fighting). Thus, as opposed to the movements of PLMS, bedpartners of these patients usually state that the patient is "fighting," "dreaming," or "thrashing" in sleep. Because REM sleep is proportionally more common in the last portion of the night, the timing of the events is also late in the sleep

---

The sleep history determines:

- Quantity of sleep.
- Timing of sleep.
- Quality of sleep.

---

period. It is typically found in older men and, if diagnosed, can be effectively treated with a long-acting benzodiazepine *(13)*. It presents one of many interesting symptoms sometimes uncovered when one begins to inquire about the night.

2.5. Daytime Function

The majority of patients with sleep disorders have impaired daytime function. The patient might report feeling fatigued or tired upon rising. Perhaps this is the single most important consequence of any sleep disorder. For example, the frustration of insomnia is probably not as critical to the patient as the subsequent daytime fatigue. The increased cardiovascular morbidity of OSA is best proven only for the most severe forms, but impaired daytime function often causes a patient to seek help and motivates one to solve the problem. Errors in the workplace or motor vehicle accidents caused by daytime sleepiness can result in tragic consequences *(14)*. Insight into the patients propensity to fall asleep during the day can be examined with a simple psychometric instrument, the Epworth Sleepiness Scale (Fig. 4) *(15)*. This questionnaire has been validated against the Multiple Sleep Latency Test (MSLT), a quantitative test of the propensity to fall asleep that is performed in the sleep laboratory. Any patient with a sleep complaint should complete the Epworth Sleepiness Scale as a rough quantitative (but subjective) measure of sleepiness. A score of under 10 can be considered normal (although 2 to 5 is probably desirable); 10 to 15 connotes moderate sleepiness and 16 to 24 severe sleepiness. Although surprising to some, it is clear that certain individuals greatly underestimate their daytime sleepiness before treatment. Thus, although important, the medical history of both sleep and sleepiness can be difficult to obtain accurately. This seems to be particularly common in sleep apnea and is most likely caused by the gradual onset of daytime impairment such that the patient loses his or her "frame of reference" for full alertness. In patients who deny significant daytime impairment, corroboration of the history by the spouse or family members is essential in excluding a disorder of excessive sleepiness.

Epworth Sleepiness Scale

Name:_____

Today's date:_____ Your age (years):_____

Your gender (male = M; female = F):_____

How likely are you to doze off or fall asleep in the following situations, in contrast to just feeling tired? This refers to your usual way of life in recent times. (Even if you have not done some of these things recently, try to work out how they would have affected you.) Use the following scale to choose the most appropriate number for each situation:

0 = Would never doze
1 = Slight chance of dozing
2 = Moderate chance of dozing
3 = High chance of dozing

Situation   **Chance of dozing**

1. Sitting and reading.   _____
2. Watching television.   _____
3. Sitting inactive in a public place (e.g., theatre).   _____
4. As a passenger in a car for an hour without a break. _____
5. Lying down to rest in the afternoon when   _____
     circumstances permit.
6. Sitting and talking to someone.   _____
7. Sitting quietly after lunch without alcohol.   _____
8. In a car, while stopped for a few minutes in traffic. _____

                                           Total score _____

Thank you for your cooperation

Fig. 4. The Epworth Sleepiness Scale. Reproduced with permission from *(15)*.

An inadequate quantity or quality of sleep virtually always results in some kind of daytime complaint. For the insomniac, the complaints are more typically tiredness, fatigue, exhaustion, or poor concentration. Many insomniacs are not sleepy in the daytime despite little sleep at night, which is consistent with a model of hyperarousal. On the other hand, most patients with significant sleep apnea or PLMS are sleepy. Usually, careful and directed questioning can distinguish the complaint of sleepiness from the complaint of fatigue. It is important to ask what happens when the patient finally gives in to the fatigue and lies down—does he or she sleep or just rest? Is the feeling mostly mental or mostly physical? Is the problem one of reasoning and focus or actual yawning and nodding off? Despite the best efforts to distinguish sleepiness from fatigue, however, many patients have both; in some, a distinction cannot be made. It is also important to stress that a distinction is not always necessary: either complaint must be taken seriously, although the complaint of sleepiness is more indicative of a nocturnal sleep-disrupting condition or narcolepsy. The patient's basal level of arousal and anxiety interacts with whatever the process of sleepiness is, however. For example, most of us have had the feeling of being both sleep-deprived and are thus sleepy, yet at the same time "wired" with difficulty falling asleep. In some cases, sleepiness such as from sleep apnea can interact with depression or anxiety to produce more complex neurocognitive dysfunction than just "sleepiness."

Headaches in the night or upon awakening can be another symptom of poor sleep and is thought to be especially indicative of OSA. Headaches that occur in the morning and are present upon awakening are most suggestive of a direct sleep–headache causal relation *(16,23)*. OSA can cause headaches directly, but it can also be a trigger for either tension-type headaches or migraines in susceptible individuals. The mechanism is not clear, but effects of hypercapnia and hypoxia on cranial vessels seems likely, or perhaps it is a neurochemical effect from disrupted sleep. Treatment of the OSA can be helpful in many types of headaches syndromes and occasionally curative.

Patients with narcolepsy may experience sudden loss of control of postural muscle tone in association with certain strong emotions such as anger, laughter, or surprise. Sometimes these events are subtle, characterized by loss of focus or weakness in the neck or knees *(12)*. This symptom, known as cataplexy, is virtually pathognomonic of narcolepsy (*see* Chapter 5). These events can be misinterpreted as seizure activity or as vertebrobasilar drop attacks. Sometimes, patients without cataplexy report frequent brief episodes of weakness, especially those with pain, myositis, and chronic fatigue, but careful questioning can usually distinguish nonspecific instances of weakness from true cataplexy.

2.6. Special Considerations

Patients who complain primarily of difficulty getting to sleep or staying asleep should be questioned about their lifestyle and sleep hygiene (Table 3). Factors impacting on sleep hygiene include: a poorly configured bedroom environment (i.e., too bright, too loud, television turned

Table 3
Sleep Hygiene

Bedroom environment
 1. Keep the bedroom environment conducive to sleep—quiet, dark, and not
    used for activities other than sleep (and sex, if applicable).
 2. Do not watch television from bed or use the bedroom to pay bills or to work.
 3. Maintain a comfortable temperature such that awakenings in the night are
    not required to open or to close windows, turn on fans, etc.
Sleep schedule
 1. The time spent in bed should be curtailed to match the actual time asleep.
 2. Arise at the same time every day.
 3. The approximate bedtime should be calculated backward from the
    wake-up time based on the expected hours of sleep.
 4. Get out of bed if not able to sleep, especially if feeling tense, angry, or
    frustrated.
 5. Limit naps to 30 minutes in the early afternoon.
Drug effects
 1. Avoid caffeine, alcohol, and tobacco, particularly after lunch.
 2. Avoid regular or frequent use of sedative-hypnotics.
 3. Assess medications for potential sleep effects.
Exercise daily
Light exposure
 1. Spend time outdoors to increase light exposure.
 2. Try to schedule the outdoor time at the same time each day.

on, a space utilized for multiple activities); an irregular sleep schedule;
and drug effects (e.g., alcohol, caffeine, and nicotine). Sleep hygiene
recommendations are discussed more completely in Chapter 2.

A frequent cause of difficulty initiating sleep is the "physiologic jet
lag" that results from sleep period being delayed on weekends. For
some, staying up late on Friday or Saturday nights and sleeping in on
Saturdays and Sundays cause a delay in the body clock that causes sleep
onset insomnia on Sunday night and difficulty awakening on Monday.
Usually, this is a trivial condition, but in some instances, it can be severe.
Shift workers are often poor sleepers. These individuals rarely adapt to
sleeping during the day; therefore they are a great risk for chronic sleep
deprivation. These problems are covered in more detail in the chapter on
circadian rhythms, but a high clinical suspicion and initial inquiry is
necessary to identify these patients.

Regular exercise has many benefits, including promoting better quality sleep (17); thus, in patients who exercise little or not at all, exercise
can be recommended. Light exposure can also affect sleep quality. In
fact, one's overall lifestyle including such factors as exercise, light

exposure, stress levels, schedules, and diet are involved in the complex function we call the "sleep-wake cycle." No single factor should be ignored, and each has a special place in any one person's sleep complaint.

3. THE PHYSICAL EXAMINATION

Because sleep and sleep quality are affected by so many variables, a complete physical examination should be performed in most patients. One of the most important aspects is the mental status examination. The physician should actively consider the possibility of a psychiatric condition in any patient with a sleep or alertness complaint. Thus, a brief assessment of the mental status is important to assess for depression, delusional thoughts, cognitive impairment, or simply unrealistic expectations. Many patients are seen each year who are referred for insomnia, for example, who turn out to have Alzheimer's disease or depression. In addition to the mental status, a brief neurologic examination should be performed to assess for signs of vascular disease (stroke) or for peripheral neuropathy—two conditions which commonly impact sleep quality.

In patients with sleep-disordered breathing, the physical examination is of utmost importance, is often abnormal and can reinforce the suspicion of sleep apnea. In the general population, obesity is a dominant risk factor, particularly upper body obesity as reflected by neck size. In men, neck sizes of greater than 42 cm, and in women, neck sizes greater than 40 cm, increase the risk for sleep apnea (7). Large necks correlate positively with narrowing of the pharyngeal airway (18). Diurnal systemic hypertension is associated with obstructive sleep-disordered breathing independent of age, sex, weight, and smoking status (6). Patients with retrognathia or midface abnormalities can develop obstructive sleep-disordered breathing without concomitant obesity. These skeletal deficiencies can be markers for a narrow pharyngeal airway. A high arched hard palate with a narrow intramaxillary intermolar distance can result in increased nasal resistance, snoring, and airway closure during sleep. In adults with untreated obstructive sleep-disordered breathing, the examination of the soft palate can reveal crowding of the tonsillar pillars with a low hanging, erythematous, and edematous soft palate. As opposed to children with sleep-disordered breathing, adults infrequently have the finding of tonsillar hypertrophy. If tonsillar hypertrophy is present, questioning regarding the chronicity of this finding should be pursued. If the tonsillar hypertrophy is new or of recent onset, infection with human immunodeficiency virus (HIV) should be considered (19). Evidence of right heart failure manifested as bilateral lower extremity edema with or without chronic venous stasis changes can be seen in

The physical examination of most patients with a sleep complaint should emphasize:

- Mental status assessment.
- Brief neurologic assessment.
- Upper airway assessment, especially the oral cavity, jaw structure, and nasal patency.
- General examination especially cardiac and pulmonary assessments.

patients with obstructive sleep-disordered breathing. Patients who are massively obese or who have concomitant obstructive lung disease are more likely to present with these physical findings.

The findings presented above are all factors that, when present, increase the likelihood of the patient having OSA. In fact, OSA is a syndrome which interacts with the patient's other systems, both mental and physical. Of primary importance is to assess for cardiovascular, pulmonary, and neurologic physical exam findings. OSA should not be treated without consideration of other conditions, for example, asthma, congestive heart failure, or stroke.

4. LABORATORY DATA

Certain laboratory findings are sometimes encountered in patients with certain sleep disorders, for example, polycythemia is occasionally seen in patients with sleep apnea. This is related to recurrent nocturnal hypoxemia, usually severe enough to produce a low mean saturation level overnight. This usually occurs in obese patients. Blood gas abnormalities (hypoxemia and hypercapnia) out of proportion to the abnormalities on spirometry can also be seen. Unexplained pulmonary hypertension by echocardiography or right heart catheterization should also suggest a diagnosis of sleep apnea *(20)*. Proteinuria has been reported in patients with OSA *(21)*.

Hypothyroidism can cause sleep apnea, but it should be remembered that thyroid replacement does not uniformly and completely correct the sleep-disordered breathing abnormality *(22)*. Patients with severe apnea should not have definitive treatment (such as nasal continuous positive airway pressure [CPAP]) withheld when hypothyroidism is being corrected. Hyperthyroidism can be a cause of fatigue or insomnia.

Patients with insomnia should undergo a routine screening of chemistries and a complete blood count. If restless legs is a specific complaint, measures of iron status and B-12 levels should be checked.

5. ASSESSMENT AND TREATMENT

Not all patients with sleep disorders require a sleep specialist consultation or sleep laboratory testing. The benefits of a careful sleep history and physical in a patient with a suspected sleep disorder are that unnecessary specialty referral and testing might be avoided and that patients with potentially life-threatening sleep disorders can be identified with confidence and promptly referred for definitive treatment. Recognition is the key issue.

5.1. Primary Problem: Difficulty Getting to Sleep or Staying Asleep

Patients who experience the primary complaint of difficulty getting to sleep or staying asleep should first be carefully assessed for proper sleep hygiene. Correcting problems with sleep hygiene (especially adding exercise, light, and decreasing time in bed) is sometimes the only intervention required. In patients with chronic pain syndromes, sleep can be substantially fragmented; thus, optimizing the pain control regimen might restore sleep continuity. Depression or anxiety can also impact negatively on sleep initiation and continuity and must be considered early. Proper treatment with antidepressants or sedatives can be curative. Nightmares and night terrors, even though infrequent, may only require reassurance as an intervention. Patients with restless leg symptoms that are not associated with significant daytime sleepiness might be given an empiric trial of a benzodiazepine prior to referral for sleep testing.

Patients with complex motor activity during sleep should in most cases be referred to a sleep specialist or a neurologist with expertise in sleep disorders. These patients frequently benefit from in laboratory sleep testing with video monitoring to characterize the parasomnia.

5.2. Primary Problem: Fatigued, Sleepy, or Tired During the Day

If insufficient sleep is identified as a factor contributing to a complaint of excessive daytime sleepiness or fatigue, sleep extension should be prescribed. Alcohol and drug use (prescribed or illicit) needs to be carefully reviewed. On occasion, an atypical depression can present with daytime sleepiness or fatigue. Hypothyriodism should be ruled out. If cataplexy is considered possible, the patient should be referred for specialist evaluation prior to the initiation of treatment. Patients with narcolepsy should probably be comanaged with a sleep specialist or a neurologist with expertise in the treatment of the disor-

der. Chronic fatigue syndrome can be an example of hypersomnolence: as many as 20% of patients with a chronic fatigue syndrome
may have occult sleep apnea.

Patients in whom the history and physical examination suggest the
diagnosis of sleep disordered breathing should be evaluated further with
an overnight sleep study. This allows the clinician to stratify the patient's
risk (*see* Chapter 6). Patients who require prompt referral to a sleep
specialist or a pulmonologist with expertise in sleep-related breathing
disorders are those individuals who report severe daytime sleepiness or
fatigue, nocturnal angina, poorly controlled systemic hypertension, or
inadequately explained blood gas abnormalities, pulmonary hypertension, or right heart failure.

A thorough evaluation for a primary disorder of daytime sleepiness is
mandatory in any patient who has had an automobile or work-related
accident related to falling asleep that is not associated with drugs, alcohol,
or sleep deprivation. The differential diagnosis of sleepiness includes
PLMS, narcolepsy, psychiatric states, neurodegenerative conditions;
many of these can only be diagnosed with sleep laboratory testing.

REFERENCES

1. Ball EM, Simon RD, Tall AA, Banks MB, Nino-Murcia G, Dement WC. Diagnosis
   and treatment of sleep apnea within the community: the Walla Walla project. *Arch
   Intern Med* 1997; 157: 419–424.
2. Rosen RC, Rosekind M, Rosevear C, Cole WE, Dement WC. Physician education
   in sleep and sleep disorders: a national survey of U.S. medical schools. *Sleep* 1993;
   16: 249–254.
3. Haponik EF, Frye AW, Richards B, et al. Sleep history is neglected information:
   challenges for the primary care physician. *J Gen Intern Med* 1996; 11: 759–761.
4. Young T, Palta M, Dempsey J, Skatrud J, Weber S, Badr S. The occurrence of sleep
   disordered breathing among middle-aged adults. *N Engl J Med* 1993; 328: 1230–1235.
5. The Gallup Organization. Sleep in America. The Gallup Organization, Princeton
   NJ, 1991.
6. Strollo PJ, Rogers RM. Obstructive sleep apnea. *N Engl J Med* 1996; 334: 99–104.
7. National Heart, Lung, and Blood Institute, Working Group on Sleep Apnea. Sleep
   apnea: is your patient at risk? *Am Fam Physician* 1996; 53: 247–253.
8. Krieger J, Laks L, Wilcox I, et al. Atrial natriuretic peptide release during sleep in
   patients with obstructive sleep apnea before and during treatment with nasal CPAP.
   Clin Sci 1989; 77: 407–411.
9. Chan HS, Chiu HF, Tse LK, Woo KS. Obstructive sleep apnea presenting with
   nocturnal angina, heart failure, and near-miss sudden death. *Chest* 1991; 99: 1023–1025.
10. Liston R, Deegan PC, McCreery C, McNicholas WT. Role of respiratory sleep
    disorders in the pathogenesis of nocturnal angina and arrhythmias. *Postgrad Med
    J* 1994; 70: 275–280.
11. Kerr P, Shoenut JP, Millar T, Buckle P, Kryger MH. Nasal CPAP reduces gas-
    troesophageal reflux in obstructive sleep apnea syndrome. *Chest* 1992; 101:
    1539–1544.

12. Aldrich MS. Narcolepsy. *N Engl J Med* 1990; 323: 389–394.
13. Schenck CH, Bundlie SR, Patterson AL, Mahowald MW. Rapid eye movement sleep behavior disorder: a treatable parasomnia affecting older adults. *JAMA* 1987; 257: 1786–1789.
14. Strohl KP (Chairman), Bonnie RJ, Findley L, et al. Sleep Apnea, Sleepiness, and Driving Risk. *Am J Respir Crit Care Med* 1994; 150: 1463–1473.
15. Johns MW. A new method for measuring daytime sleepiness: the Epworth Sleepiness Scale. *Sleep* 1991; 14: 540–545.
16. Aldrich MS, Chauncey JB. Are morning headaches part of obstructive sleep apnea syndrome? *Arch Intern Med* 1991; 150: 1265–1267.
17. King AC, Oman RF, Brassington GS, Bliwise DL, Haskell WL. Moderate-intensity exercise and self-rated quality of sleep in older adults. *JAMA* 1997; 277: 32–37.
18. Davies RJO, Stradling JR. The relationship between neck circumference, radiographic pharyngeal anatomy, and the obstructive sleep apnea syndrome. *Eur Respir J* 1990; 3: 509–514.
19. Epstein LJ, Strollo PJ, Donegan RB, Delmar J, Hendrix C, Westbrook PR. Obstructive sleep apnea in patients with human immunodeficiency virus (HIV) disease. *Sleep* 1995; 18: 368–376.
20. Weitzenblum E, Krieger J, Apprill M, et al. Daytime pulmonary hypotension in patients with obstructive sleep apnea syndrome. *Am Rev Respir Dis* 1988; 138: 345–349.
21. Chaudhary BA, Sklar AH, Chaudhary TK, Kolbeck RC, Speir WA. Sleep apnea, proteinuria, and nephrotic syndrome. *Sleep* 1988; 11: 69–74.
22. Grunstein RR, Sullivan CE. Hypothyroidism and sleep apnea: mechanisms and management. *Am J Med* 1988; 85: 775–779.
23. Poceta JS, Dalessio DJ. Identification and treatment of obstructive sleep apnea in patients with chronic headache. *Headache* 1995; 35: 586–589.
24. Kryger M, Roth T, Dement W. *Principles and practice of sleep medicine.* W.B. Saunders, Philadelphia, 1994.

2 Insomnia

Milton K. Erman

CONTENTS

1. INTRODUCTION

Insomnia is the most common sleep complaint both in the general population and in various medical and psychiatric patient populations. Studies in recent years have shown typical prevalence rates of about one-third in randomly selected adult populations. For example, a recent Gallup poll found that almost one-half of adult Americans complained of disturbed sleep, with 35% reporting this as a problem "only at certain times" and an additional 12% stating that this was a problem "on a frequent basis." Women and adults under 35 years of age comprised populations more likely to complain of insomnia.

What defines insomnia as a medical problem? Can we be certain that the presence of these complaints reflects a "disease" state that should be of concern to patients and physicians, or do the differences that patients report in sleep duration and sleep quality represent differences in sleep capacity or perception of sleep quality that should not necessarily be considered a medical problem? In this chapter, before attempting to

From: *Sleep Disorders: Diagnosis and Treatment*
Edited by: J. S. Poceta and M. M. Mitler © Humana Press Inc., Totowa, NJ

define insomnia and to discuss its development and treatment, certain key questions will be addressed. Why do we sleep? How much sleep do we need? What are the health and performance consequences of insufficient sleep?

1.1. Why Do We Sleep?

The answers to this age-old question may range from the complex to the simple. Complex responses may invoke reviews of phylogeny, energy expenditure, and hypotheses regarding brain development, memory storage, the need for repair and nutrition of brain and body, and so forth. At a more practical level, we sleep to reverse the negative effects of extended periods of wakefulness on the body and brain and to restore the metabolic capability of neurons, or even more simply, we sleep because we feel so terrible when we do not.

From an evolutionary perspective, it is obvious that sleep plays a critical role in physiology. Were it not an element essential for survival, classes of animals as diverse as mammals, birds, amphibians, reptiles, fish, and even insects would not "waste time" (and be left defenseless to predators) sleeping for a substantial portion of their life cycles. Animals with more time available in each 24-hour cycle to hunt, feed, and procreate should be able to dominate the gene pool within a species relative to "weaker" members, those requiring more sleep and thus less capable of engaging in these activities insuring survival of their lineage. Consequently, it is obvious that the evolutionary advantage of sleep is in balance with the advantage of activity. The robust and ubiquitous persistence of the "behavior" of sleep across a range of organisms from moths to man argues for its significance and physiologic necessity.

1.2. Sleep Needs

How much sleep do we need? It is often assumed by the lay public, as well as by some medical professionals, that "everyone" needs eight hours of sleep per night, that we spend (and in some people's minds, waste) a third of our lives in bed, asleep. In fact, the amount of sleep required varies greatly from individual to individual, and the amount that each of us requires is probably determined in part by heredity. Rare individuals can function well on as little as five hours of sleep on a regular basis; others may need as many as eleven hours sleep per night, an amount which may be difficult to obtain on a regular basis as a working adult. However, the vast majority of people require between 6 and 10 hours of sleep, and those requiring more or less probably can be considered abnormal. Within this range, most individuals who are given the opportunity to sleep for as long as they feel they need will sleep

To determine whether a patient is obtaining too little sleep, the patient should be directed to set aside a two-week period free of excessive responsibilities, and to:

- Eliminate caffeine and alcohol;
- Follow sleep hygiene techniques;
- Go to bed and get up from bed about 8 hours apart;
- Go to bed when sleepy, even if earlier than the scheduled bedtime;
- Get up at about the same time each morning.

If the patient is able to obtain adequate amounts of sleep in this period, he or she should be fully alert and functional throughout the day, with only mild sleepiness in a sedentary condition in the afternoon.

between seven and nine hours per night. In the absence of a primary sleep disorder, an individual who has obtained sufficient amounts of sleep should be able to remain alert and fully functional in even the most boring and tedious setting.

1.3. Sleep Deprivation

What are the health and performance consequences of insufficient sleep? Various sources of data support a hypothesis that inadequate sleep has negative health impact. Experiments performed by Dr. Alan Rechtschaffen at the University of Chicago have shown that in rats, total sleep deprivation will lead to death or to a moribund state within a period of days to weeks. This precipitous decline in health was not seen in control animals, which were subjected to the same levels of physical activity as a stressor, but who were allowed to sleep when sedentary. In humans, the direct results of extended total sleep deprivation are impossible to assess in any ethical manner, although periods of sleep deprivation of up to about 11 days have been studied. As might be expected, substantial decreases in mood, alertness, and performance were seen.

Partial sleep deprivation of even moderate severity will lead to decreases in performance and mood, a phenomenon which virtually everyone has experienced in the context of work demands, travel, or illness. Research supports this perception of the impact of inadequate sleep on human physiology. Studies performed by Dr. Michael Irwin at the University of California, San Diego, have shown the effect on immune function of impaired sleep in healthy young adults. With even a single night of partial sleep deprivation, reductions are seen in T-cell cytokine production and in killer cell numbers and their levels of activity. Several epidemiological studies of sleep and mortality have shown that lowest mortality rates exist for individuals reporting sleep times of seven to eight hours per night, and higher mortality among shorter or longer sleepers.

1.4. Costs of Insomnia

Besides medical and psychological well-being, insomnia impacts on individuals and society in other ways. The National Commission on Sleep Disorders Research of the NIH estimates that the direct costs of insomnia in the United States, including costs of prescription medication, over-the-counter medications, alcohol used to promote sleep, and medical treatment for insomnia exceed $15 billion annually. Estimates of the total annual costs related to insomnia, including decreased productivity, health and property costs related to accidents, and medical costs from comorbid conditions, range from $30 billion (conservative) to as high as $108 billion (probably excessive). These costs include expenses related to institutionalization of elderly individuals with sleep problems, as this is a frequent and significant factor leading to the decision to place elderly individuals, especially males, in institutional settings.

These various medical and social research findings should sensitize us to the impact of insomnia on society to the concerns about the health consequences of poor sleep expressed by patients with chronic insomnia. We might even be able to begin to understand their fear, which is sometimes expressed in the throes of severe insomnia, that "Without a good night's sleep" they will soon surely die. Perhaps paradoxically, despite the concerns, excessive anxiety over insomnia is counterproductive for the patient, and alleviating anxiety about insomnia is often part of the therapeutic process, as discussed later in this chapter.

2. DEFINING INSOMNIA

Insomnia may be thought of both as a symptom complex and a disorder, with different patients manifesting different dimensions of the problem, or with the same patient experiencing variable severity at different points in time. As a symptom, insomnia reflects the perception of inadequate sleep duration, continuity, or quality, or of difficulty with sleep initiation. These complaints are very idiosyncratic—one patient may state that he has no problems with sleep initiation—always asleep within 30–60 minutes; but a latency to sleep onset of 30 minutes to another patient may seem an eternity. Patients may report that their sleep difficulty may always occur at sleep onset, or in the middle or later hours of the night, or may be disturbed in a variable pattern that is unpredictable.

All insomnia disorders require the presence of not only night time complaints, but also daytime symptoms, such as:

- Being unrefreshed or unrestored in the morning or through the day.
- Feeling fatigued or sleepy in the day.
- Having poor concentration or attention during the day.
- Having other neuro-cognitive complaints that affect daytime performance.

2.1. Insomnia Complaints and Insomnia Disorders

When does a complaint become a disorder? Specific diagnostic criteria categories of primary insomnia and other sleep disorders are included in the Diagnostic and Statistical Manual (DSM IV) of the American Psychiatric Association. The International Classification of Sleep Disorders (ICSD), published by the American Sleep Disorders Association, is a much more extensive and well-annotated system of diagnostic classification that is specific for sleep disorders. Although the two systems differ in focus and degree of detail, one important element is common to both: to establish a diagnosis of insomnia, the disorder must lead to distress or impairment in one of several areas of daytime functioning. A complaint also does not become a diagnosable insomnia disorder until it has been present for a duration of at least a month. Terminology and diagnostic criteria used in this chapter are based on the ICSD.

2.2. Prevalence and Significance of Insomnia

As is noted above, insomnia is a very common disorder. Almost one-half of adult Americans reported disturbed sleep "sometimes or often." That these rates of prevalence should seem high to practitioners dealing with ambulatory populations is understandable, since in an earlier Gallup poll, only about 5% of patients who experienced insomnia on a chronic basis reported that they had gone to a doctor specifically seeking help for the problem.

Why should this be? Perhaps chronic insomnia is trivial and not worthy of our concern, since patients do not seek care for their symptoms. However, the Gallup polls, as well as numerous other studies, have demonstrated that mood and daytime performance are negatively influenced by insomnia and poor quality sleep. Gallup data showed that patients with insomnia report significantly impaired concentration during the day, have greater difficulty coping with minor irritations, experience a reduced ability to enjoy family and social relationships, and were even 2.5 times more likely than noninsomniacs to report having had a fatigue-related automobile accident. Patients with insomnia are more likely to report poor health and to experience fatigue and depression. Studies have also demonstrated that comparatively poor sleepers are less likely to be given promotions in work settings, are more likely to have frequent visits to their doctors for complaints not related to sleep, and are more likely to be absent from work. Thus, there must be other reasons for patient reluctance to report sleep complaints.

The Gallup poll data suggest that patients who suffer from these problems are not sure that they are significant, despite the discomfort and dysfunction they experience. Beyond this, patients are not certain that their doctor has anything to offer as help for their sleep problem, or, particularly in view of the financial constraints impacting on heath care delivery, they may feel that their doctor will not have the time to discuss it with them. Patients are self-conscious about insomnia complaints, "knowing" that if they lived more healthy life styles, ate better, exercised more, and drank less coffee and alcohol, they would sleep better and not need to burden their doctor with this problem.

Finally, for certain patients, the treatment may be more frightening than the disease. When the word "sleeping pill" is mentioned as a possible treatment, the term evokes images of well-known suicides and overdoses, from Marilyn Monroe to Judy Garland to the Heaven's Gate cult. Patients are concerned about the risks of dependency and addiction associated with the use of sleeping pills, and are unaware that the newest generation of hypnotic agents, the benzodiazepines and benzodiazepine-agonist compounds, are more effective and far safer than their antecedents in almost every category, even when taken in intentional overdose.

2.3. Insomnia in the Elderly

Insomnia and associated nocturnal behavioral disturbances are a particular problem in elderly populations. These problems are more difficult for family and caregivers to manage in the home than are many other geriatric disabilities. In one large study, insomnia was the most important predictor of institutionalization for elderly men and the most important mortality predictor. A British study of caregivers' reasons for institutionalization of a family member revealed that "sleep disturbance" was the most cited problem and was mentioned by 62% of cases. This reason was also highly ranked as one that, if alleviated, would allow for the patient to return home.

Potential causes of insomnia include:

- External factors, such as a travel schedule or drug use.
- Psychiatric conditions, such as depression or anxiety.
- Medical conditions, such as pain or Parkinson's Disease.
- Specific sleep disorders, such as restless legs syndrome, circadian phase problem, or sleep apnea.
- "Intrinsic" problems, such as conditioned insomnia.

---

3. CAUSES OF INSOMNIA COMPLAINTS

Insomnia complaints may be the primary complaint in many sleep disorders, including extrinsic sleep disorders, which are sleep disturbances which develop as a result of factors or forces outside the body, and circadian rhythm sleep disorders. Some common examples of these types of disorders are discussed below. Although these disorders are relatively easily understood and easily treated when they are recognized, they may also lead to the development of more sustained problems if untreated. That is, virtually all psychophysiological insomnias begin with in initiating factor that might be minor, and become established on a more chronic basis as a result of arousal and conditioning factors.

3.1. Extrinsic Insomnia Disorders

3.1.1. JET LAG

Jet lag, a circadian rhythm sleep disorder, is dealt with in detail in Chapter 3. It may serve as a conceptual model for extrinsic sleep disorders, since it occurs in response to an external factor—transmeridian (East-West) travel. This disorder is characterized by complaints of insomnia, altered sleep/wake schedules and/or excessive sleepiness, and is almost universally experienced after rapid travel across multiple time zones.

3.1.2. ADJUSTMENT SLEEP DISORDER

Adjustment sleep disorder is another form of sleep disturbance which virtually all adults have experienced. This disorder reflects a change from typical sleep patterns and occurs as a result of stress, conflict, or environmental change causing emotional arousal. This disorder is typically seen during periods of interpersonal or intrapsychic conflict, preceding major life changes (i.e., marriage, divorce, birth of a child), in the course of intense job or career demands or following sudden disappointments and frightening events. The stress may also result from "normal" developmental events, such as the start of the school year or week, school examinations, family or financial conflicts, and so forth. When the stressor remits, the patient will usually quickly return to normal patterns of sleep.

A patient with this disorder will often have a prior history of normal sleep. The insomnia may recur when the susceptible individual again experiences a high level of stress. This usually unambiguous real sleep disturbance may be viewed as an "insomnia of everyday life,"—expected and predictable, considering the diverse stresses we face over the course of a lifetime. However, an individual who is insecure or vulnerable to emotional arousal is most frequently and severely affected. In this person, the frequency and severity of sleep disruption can reach the level of a serious clinical problem that requires intervention. For this person also, an adjustment sleep disorder may initiate negative conditioning that can precipitate and propagate a chronic problem.

3.1.3. INADEQUATE SLEEP HYGIENE

In this condition, the patient engages in practices and habits that are under his or her behavioral control and that cause arousal or disrupt sleep rhythms. Examples of arousing stimuli would include exercising too late in the day (i.e., too close to bedtime), engaging in intense mental activity late at night, consuming excessive amounts of caffeine or cigarettes near bedtime, or allowing the bedroom to be too light, too noisy, or excessively hot or cold. Examples of behaviors which can disrupt sleep rhythms would include large day-to-day variation in sleep schedules, spending excessive time in bed, or daytime napping.

3.1.4. DRUG AND ALCOHOL USE

An important cause of insomnia complaints is chronic hypnotic drug use, as first described by Kales and associates. The sleep disturbance of patients on chronic drug regimens (months to years) may be exacerbated by the medication use itself. However, if medications are abruptly stopped, the resulting withdrawal syndrome further disturbs sleep. In a similar fashion, withdrawal from alcohol or anti-anxiety agents may also lead to insomnia.

This disturbance is far more likely to be seen with the barbiturate and barbiturate-like drugs than with benzodiazepine and benzodiazepine-agonist compounds. However, a drug-rebound insomnia can occur with short and ultrashort half-life benzodiazepine agents, such as triazolam, especially when used in higher doses.

Another important cause of insomnia is stimulant use or abuse. Illicit stimulant drug use can obviously lead to a disturbance of this sort, as can excessive ingestion of tea, coffee, or caffeine-containing over-the-counter stimulants. Legal restrictions and changes in medical practice have limited the extent to which stimulant compounds such as the amphetamines and methylphenidate are now prescribed, but other less tightly controlled compounds are still widely used. Excessive use or abuse of these agents can obviously also lead to psychomotor stimulation and insomnia complaints. The widespread use of these compounds necessitates consideration of this as a source of insomnia complaints in all patients, even those for whom this may seem unlikely or improbable.

3.1.5. MEDICAL CONDITIONS

Insomnia complaints can develop as a result of several types of medical problems. Any source of somatic pain or physical discomfort from conditions as diverse as arthritis, metastatic disease, pruritis, nocturia, or the effects of trauma or surgery can lead to disturbed sleep. Cardiac disturbances can lead to symptoms of angina or paroxysmal nocturnal dyspnea; pulmonary disorders such as chronic obstructive pulmonary disease, cystic fibrosis, and hypoventilation secondary to polio, paralysis or scoliosis can produce drops in oxygenation, arousal, and disturbed sleep. Other organic causes include endocrine disorders such as hyperthyroidism and hypoglycemia, gastroesophageal reflux, and renal disease.

3.2. Intrinsic Insomnia Disorders

Intrinsic sleep disorders are those sleep disturbances that originate or develop within the body or arise from causes within the body. Among causes of insomnia that are defined as intrinsic in origin are psychophysiological insomnia, idiopathic insomnia, periodic limb movement disorder, and restless legs syndrome.

3.2.1. ACUTE (TRANSIENT) PSYCHOPHYSIOLOGICAL INSOMNIA

Psychophysiological insomnia is the insomnia condition seen most frequently in general patient populations. This acute or transient category refers to sleep disturbances of up to one month in duration. These disturbances may initially be provoked by jet lag or brief hospitalizations; they may arise as well from emotional arousal or conflict caused by any type of loss or perceived threat. The disturbances may present with any combination of sleep complaints such as difficulty falling asleep, intermittent awakenings, and premature early morning arousal (most notable when a depressive component is present).

This disturbance develops in association with negative conditioning to sleep and the sleep environment. The patients become more anxious as bedtime approaches, and will often "try too hard" to fall asleep, increasing the level of arousal and anxiety and further diminishing the ability to fall asleep. They are afraid to get up from bed for fear of "really waking up", and become more frustrated lying in bed, awake, establishing negative associations between the bed, the bedroom, and the ability to sleep. The common awareness that insomnia has a tendency to "feed on itself" fits well with a conditioning model.

As confidence in the ability to sleep decreases and apprehension about poor sleeping increases, the insomnia may become persistent and take on "a life of its own." The patient develops a virtual neurosis about the process of sleeping. This can lead to the development of subacute or chronic psychophysiological insomnia.

3.2.2. SUBACUTE AND CHRONIC PSYCHOPHYSIOLOGICAL INSOMNIA

This condition is diagnosed when the insomnia complaints have been present for one to six months in duration (subacute), or for longer than six months (chronic). The chronic form most typically has been present for many months or years before the patient is evaluated by a physician interested in sleep disorders. The conditioning component of this insomnia is an independent element that may become attached to almost any other cause of insomnia, including psychiatric disturbances. This process constitutes the mechanism of long-term entrenchment of insomnia.

The hallmark of this insomnia syndrome is the focused absorption of the patient on the sleep problem itself. The patient tends to minimize other mental and emotional concerns. He or she usually demonstrates good family and work relationships and competent daily functioning, not the general maladaptive behavior of the conventional psychiatric patient.

These patients continually make great efforts to sleep when lying in bed, unaware of the effect of this effort in leading to arousal. They become increasingly anxious about sleep and develop a negative expectation (an internal conditioning factor) about sleeping in their own bedrooms. The bedroom, which is an external conditioning factor, thus becomes associated with difficulty in sleeping, and the patient paradoxically sleeps better in other rooms of the house and/or away from his or her home. A patient with chronic psychophysiological insomnia often sleeps better in the sleep laboratory than at home, an experience that can be embarrassing, as the patient might assume the staff will not believe he or she really has a sleep problem. However, this patient is usually quite accurate in estimates of sleep latency and sleep duration, and sleeps better in this "abnormal" setting where not expecting to sleep and thus relieved of the need to try so hard to fall asleep.

The patient with psychophysiological insomnia typically reports having no idea why he or she does not sleep. This is because conditioning factors responsible for poor sleep are not obvious or intuitive. The tendency not to sleep, however, emerges every time the patient is again in a situation associated with earlier sleep difficulties. The diagnosis of persistent psychophysiological insomnia should be used when insomnia-reinforcing mechanisms (i.e., apprehensive overconcern about sleep) are strongly represented in the patient's history.

3.2.3. RESTLESS LEGS SYNDROME AND PERIODIC LIMB MOVEMENT DISORDER

These relatively common causes of insomnia are reviewed in detail in Chapter 4. They are more common in older patient populations. Many individuals with periodic limb movement disorder may be asymptomatic, but spouses or bedpartners often report being kicked at night or having their sleep otherwise disturbed by the repetitive movements. Patients with these movement disorders are at increased risk of psychophysiologic conditioned insomnia as well.

3.2.4. SLEEP APNEA

Sleep apnea disorders are covered in detail in Chapter 6. Although sleep apnea is far more likely to be associated with complaints of excessive sleepiness, it can present with insomnia complaints. It should be considered when patients report awakenings of unclear origin multiple times per night but no major problems at sleep onset or with the capacity to return to sleep during the night, and in patients whose primary complaint is nonrestorative sleep and daytime fatigue.

3.2.5. PSYCHIATRIC DISTURBANCES

Psychiatric patients comprise a population very much at risk for experiencing insomnia. The specific changes in sleep physiology associated with seasonal affective disorders are discussed in Chapter 3. The specific sleep findings of depression have been of interest on both clinical and research grounds. These abnormalities include sleep continuity disturbances, diminished slow-wave sleep, an abbreviated first nonREM sleep period leading to the early appearance of the first REM sleep period, and altered intranight distribution of REM sleep, with increased REM time and activity in the first half of the night. Despite the long-held belief that these findings were specific to affective disorders and might be understood in some context as relating to intrapsychic origins of depression, it has now been well demonstrated that sleep in patients with schizophrenia and schizoaffective illness is indistinguishable on objective grounds from that of patients with depression.

From a clinical perspective, the report of changes in sleep habits often serves to alert the clinician to the possibility that depression may be present. These patients often complain of early morning awakening, disturbed midnocturnal sleep, or delayed sleep onset. Although most depressed patients report a decrease in overall sleep time, a smaller number report increased sleep time and daytime sleepiness. These hypersomniac complaints are more likely to be reported by patients in the depressed phase of bipolar affective disorder.

3.2.6. MANIA

The sleep disturbance in mania, with marked decreases in total sleep time and time in bed, is also well described. Manic patients, however, often deny or are unaware that such changes have occurred. Manic patients may feel quite well when sleeping only four or five hours per night for long periods of time, but most are aware of the changed sleep patterns and are often eager to describe it. As part of the general psychiatric history, particularly where affective illness is suspected, it is thus helpful to ask a spouse, family member, or roommate about changes in the patient's sleeping habits.

3.2.7. SCHIZOPHRENIA

Acute schizophrenia is also associated with a sleep disturbance, marked by delayed sleep onset, decreased total sleep time, and increased time awake after sleep onset. Although considerable interest has been expressed for many years about the possibility that schizophrenic hallucinations might be associated with abnormalities in REM sleep, no consistent findings reflecting this hypothesis have been described.

3.2.8. INSOMNIA AND DEPRESSION

The relationship between insomnia and depression is complicated by the fact that there appears to be a causal interaction between the two disorders: insomnia is associated with (and likely causative of) depression; depression produces insomnia, often as an early sign or "harbinger of things to come." As has been shown in a number of studies, including the Epidemiologic Catchment Area survey by Ford and Kamerow, the presence of insomnia on a persistent basis for a period of greater than a year is associated with increases in risk of depression. This causal relationship seems inherently obvious to our patients: when they do not sleep (or sleep poorly), they feel depressed; when they sleep well, their mood is improved. If they have a predisposition to clinical depression, their extended sleep deprivation may precipitate an episode of "serious" or "major" depression.

Although this intimate relationship is important to understand, it must be remembered that not all insomnia are caused by depression, even when some depressive complaints are seen in association with the complaint of insomnia. Similarly, the fact that symptoms of insomnia may be effectively treated by use of a low dose antidepressant does not imply or suggest that the insomnia complaint is caused by depression. Other causes should be considered and explored.

4. TAKING AN INSOMNIA HISTORY

To provide effective and appropriate treatment in any medical specialty, physicians must be able to make an accurate diagnosis. As with any diagnostic dilemma, data is gathered from a patient interview, from medical records (if available) and from a physical and mental examination of the patient. If they plan to care for insomniac patients, physicians must know the elements of a sleep history, as well as diagnostic criteria for the major sleep disorders.

Unfortunately, the limited training received in medical school regarding sleep (typically less than two hours over four years) and the limited formal training about Sleep Medicine provided in most residency training programs leaves even the interested and motivated physician with a "knowledge gap" that is hard to fill.

Table 1 presents a series of questions that might be asked in a "sleep history." These questions probe the patient's expectations about sleep and define the perception of the sleep problem. They address issues regarding the patient's sleep schedule and sleep habits, as well to be able to provide information regarding possible primary sleep disorders (i.e., apnea, periodic limb movements) and elements of poor sleep hygiene that may disrupt sleep quality or continuity. Further information on taking a "sleep history" is presented in Chapter 1.

Figure 1 is a schematic diagram of the considerations in creating a differential diagnosis for a patient with insomnia. The diagram emphasizes certain key historical information in formulating a working diagnosis and then beginning treatment.

5. TREATMENT OF INSOMNIA

Insomnia usually develops as a consequence and combination of disturbances in habits, circadian rhythm, mood, and underlying sleep physiology. Effective treatment requires that these individual contributing factors be identified and, where possible, addressed separately in treatment. Although behavioral management must always be included in the management strategy for the insomniac patient, pharmacotherapy is often needed as well, at times combined with behavioral treatment.

Table 1
Elements of a Brief Insomnia History

1. What is the specific insomnia complaint—sleep initiation, sleep maintenance, early awakening, or nonrestorative sleep?
2. What is the subjective perception of sleep quality? Is it sound, restorative? What are the patient's attitudes towards sleep?
3. How much sleep is needed on a daily basis to feel alert and energetic when awake? How often is that amount of sleep obtained? What are daytime symptoms related to poor sleep?
4. What is the schedule of retiring and rising? Is there variation between weekdays and weekends? Have there been recent changes in the sleep–wake schedule?
5. How does the patient use caffeine and alcohol?
6 Is snoring present? If so, with what severity and frequency? Are leg movements or other disturbances present in sleep?
7. Are there general emotional or medical problems? How are they treated? What medications does the patient use?
8. What is the sleep environment like, including temperature, bed comfort, noise, and light?

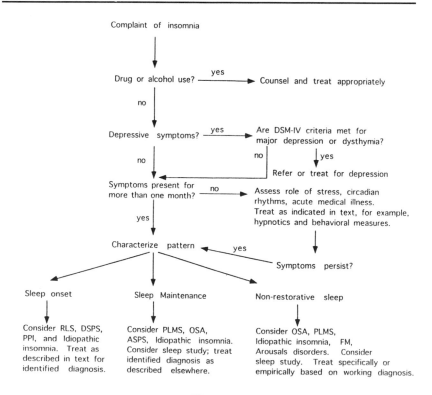

Fig. 1.

5.1. Behavioral Treatments of Insomnia

Many approaches to insomnia are based on the observation that insomniac patients are tense, anxious, or excessively aroused. Various strategies can be used to combat this state of excessive arousal; among these are progressive relaxation techniques, self-hypnosis, meditation, abdominal breathing, biofeedback, and a host of other similar approaches.

5.1.1. Stimulus Control Therapy

A specific treatment approach to insomnia is stimulus control therapy, developed by Bootzin. This approach is based on the hypothesis that the sleep environment has become associated with a state of greater arousal specific to presleep factors, as demonstrated in the complaint often heard from insomniac patients that they are able to fall asleep in the living room, but not in their bedroom. In order to break this conditioned pattern of association, patients are given specific rules to follow that encourage only sleep-promoting behaviors in the bedroom. Many of the components of this specific approach are included in published lists of "Do's and Don't's" that insomniacs should follow in order to obtain better sleep; a complete description and explanation of this approach appears in Table 2.

5.1.2. Sleep Restriction Therapy

Another behavioral-derived approach is that of sleep restriction therapy. This technique, developed by Spielman, is based on the recognition that excessive time spent in bed is an important factor in the development and perpetuation of insomnia. By limiting time spent in bed, more efficient sleep ensues. This improvement in sleep efficiency is also driven by a component of sleep deprivation inherent in this approach. Sleep is consolidated, and sleep patterns become more regular and predictable. Total time in bed is allowed to increase as the patient demonstrates a continuing ability to sleep in an efficient and consolidated fashion.

Fig. 1. *(previous page)* Evaluation of the complaint of insomnia. This diagram conceptualizes some of the considerations in the differential diagnosis of the insomnia complaint, and in formulating a working diagnosis so that appropriate treatment can be started. RLS is restless legs syndrome, DSPS is delayed sleep phase syndrome, ASPS is advanced sleep phase syndrome, PPI is psychophysiologic insomnia, FM is fibromyalgia. Treatment is not covered, but should be tailored to the working diagnosis, and if response is inadequate, the diagnosis should be reconsidered. Behavioral treatment can be recommended to help multiple types of insomnia, in addition to other specific treatments.

Table 2
Stimulus Control Instructions

"Rules" patients must follow
   1. Lie down intending to go to sleep only when you feel sleepy.
   2. Do not use your bed for anything except sleep; that is, do not read, watch television, eat, or worry in bed. Sexual activity is the only exception to this rule. When the bed is used for sexual activity near bedtime, the instructions are to be followed afterward when you intend to go to sleep.
   3. If you find yourself unable to fall asleep, get up and go into another room. Stay up as long as you wish, and then return to the bedroom to sleep. Although we do not want you to watch the clock, we want you to get out of bed if you do not fall asleep immediately. Remember that the goal is to associate your bed with falling asleep quickly! If you are in bed more than about ten minutes without falling asleep and have not gotten up, you are not following this instruction.
   4. If you still cannot fall asleep, repeat rule 3. Do this as often as is necessary throughout the night.
   5. Set your alarm and get up at the same time every morning irrespective of how much sleep you had during the night. This will help your body to establish consistent sleep rhythms.
   6. Do not nap during the day.

Rationales are provided to the patients to explain the function of each rule.
   1. This rule is intended to help patients become more sensitive to internal cues of sleepiness so that they will be more likely to fall asleep quickly when they go to bed.
   2. The goal of this rule is to have activities that are associated with arousal occur elsewhere and to break up patterns that are associated with disturbed sleep. If patients report that bedtime is when they think about the day's events and plan for the next day, they should do this in a quiet fashion in another room before they go to bed. Although many people without sleep problems can read or listen to music in bed without problems, that is not the case for most insomniacs. This instruction is intended to help insomniacs establish new routines to facilitate entry into sleep.
   3. To associate the bed and bedroom with sleep and disassociate them from the frustration and arousal of not being able to sleep, patients are instructed to get out of bed after about ten minutes (20 minutes for those over 60 years of age). This is also a means of coping with insomnia. By getting out of bed and engaging in other activities, patients are exerting control over their problems. The problems become more manageable; consequently, less distress is experienced. The goal is to re-associate the act of lying down in bed with falling asleep.
   4. Insomniacs often have irregular sleep schedules. They may try to make up for poor sleep by sleeping late, by taking an afternoon nap the day after a poor night's sleep, or by going to bed early the next evening to try to get more sleep. Establishing a consistent wake time helps patients develop

Table 2 *(continued)*

stable sleep rhythms, helping them to be able to fall asleep at night. Additionally, the set wake time means that patients will be somewhat sleep-deprived after a night of insomnia. This will make it more likely that they will fall asleep quickly the following night, strengthening the associations between the bed/bedroom and the capacity to sleep.

5. Insomniacs disrupt their sleep patterns by napping on an irregular schedule. A nap will also interfere with night-time sleep by decreasing sleepiness that would otherwise promote entry into sleep. If the patient is aware that an afternoon nap may make prolong wakefulness at bedtime, and that if this is a desirable effect, such as in the elderly who tend to advanced sleep phase, than a regular, daily nap may be permissible. For those elderly insomniacs who feel they need to nap, either a daily nap of less than an hour's length, or the use of 20 to 30 minutes of relaxation as a nap substitute should be suggested. The timing should only be in the period about eight hours after the morning get-up time.

An element of sleep restriction is also present in stimulus control therapy treatment owing to reduction in time in bed, and this appears to contribute to the efficacy of this technique. In sleep restriction therapy, this reduction in time in bed is acknowledged as an important part of the therapy. Thus, if the insomnia patient states that he or she has only been obtaining only five hours sleep per night despite spending eight hours in bed, the patient is instructed to spend only five hours in bed until it becomes apparent that the sleep obtained is perceived to have been consolidated. Each morning, the patient estimates how much of the five hour period he or she slept, and the patient and physician calculate "sleep efficiency," which is number of minutes asleep divided by the number of minutes in bed. When the sleep efficiency is high—at least 75%, the patient is allowed to spend 15 more minutes in bed. Five days later, the calculations are done again, and the time in bed adjusted. If the sleep efficiency is low, the time in bed is decreased, or remains the same (Table 3). This therapy requires a motivated patient and physician staff and is not usually effective simply by handing the patient a pamphlet on the therapy. However, effective results have been proven when a concerted effort is made.

5.1.3. SLEEP HYGIENE

"Sleep hygiene" refers to relatively neutral suggestions for improving sleep that are of benefit to virtually all patients with sleep problems. There is no single list that is perfect for every patient, however, and this volume contains mention to sleep hygiene activities in several chapters.

Table 3
Instructions for Sleep Restriction Therapy

1. Stay in bed for the average total subjective sleep time reported in sleep diary during the prior two weeks, plus 15 minutes, but never less than four and a half hours. For example, if total sleep time is five-and-three-quarters hours, patients are allowed to stay in bed for six hours.
2. Get up at same time each day. If normal final awakening time is 6:00 AM, one should always get up at 6:00 AM and go to bed at midnight.
3. No naps allowed during the day.
4. Call in (either to a person or to a telephone answering machine) each day to report time to bed, out-of-bed and estimated total sleep time.
5. When sleep efficiency has reached 75% over the last five days, allowed to go to bed 15 minutes earlier.
6. Procedure repeated until the patient can sleep for eight hours or desired amount of time.

For example, although most patients will benefit from an instruction to avoid naps, some patients may find that a brief nap in the afternoon may allow them an increased level of alertness and energy through the evening hours without interfering with the capacity to fall asleep at their desired bedtime hours. Also, although most patients may need to discontinue entirely use of caffeine in any form, some patients may find that caffeinated coffee or tea in the morning provides a helpful "pick-me-up" without interfering with night time sleep. Therapeutic strategies may include tactics such as regularization of the daily sleep and waking schedule, not spending time in bed if sleep remains elusive, initiating a regular exercise routine, and so forth. Establishing regular bedtimes and awakening times will help to diminish the tendency for the insomniac to spend too much time in bed "trying to sleep," a pattern that lowers sleep efficiency and leads to increased frustration and complaints.

Patients should be instructed to try to implement one or two sleep hygiene rules at a time, with instructions to monitor their progress over the period until the next office visit. They should also be aware that the effect of these types of changes produce gradual rather than dramatic improvement. One must expect continuing improvement in the regularity and depth of sleep rather than an immediate cure of their insomnia. Sleep hygiene rules are listed in Table 4.

5.1.4. REDUCTION IN ALCOHOL USE

Many people are not aware that alcohol can disrupt sleep. This potential role of alcohol as a factor that can disrupt sleep must be pointed out to some insomniacs who use alcohol in the evening hours or at bedtime,

Table 4
Sleep Hygiene Instructions

1. Sleep only as much as you need to feel refreshed in the daytime.
2. A regular exercise program in the morning or afternoon may help to promote sleep.
3. Limit alcohol intake, especially in the evening (after dinner).
4. Avoid caffeine use, especially in the late afternoon or evening.
5. Try to set aside time in the evening—at least an hour before bedtime—to deal with problems or thoughts that you have on your mind. Write down plans to cope with problems the next day—do not let them fester.
6. A light bedtime snack may help sustain sleep.
7. Keep your bedroom as dark and quiet as possible. Maintain it at a comfortable temperature.
8. If you cannot sleep and feel yourself getting more frustrated as you remain awake, get up from bed, go to another room and do something relaxing, such as reading or listening to the radio or a relaxation tape. When you feel sleepy go back to bed and go to sleep.
9. If you wake up during the night do not look at the clock: try to just "roll over and go back to sleep."
10. Your wake up time must be regular and the same on weekends as weekdays.
11. No daytime naps. These will only decrease your level of sleepiness at night and decrease the number of hours of sleep you may expect to obtain.
12. Do not worry about or focus on the number of hours of sleep you are obtaining at night. Focus instead on your level of daytime alertness and functioning. If this level is good (or at least improving) you are getting at least an adequate amount of sleep during the night.

dispelling the notion that a nightcap is a harmless and effective way to overcome sleep-initiation problems. These individuals should be instructed to decrease or completely stop alcohol consumption, especially in the evening hours or at bedtime. Incorporation of a regular exercise routine may be a helpful replacement, as might be training in biofeedback, relaxation, meditation, or self-hypnosis.

5.1.5. MEDICAL DISORDERS AND PRIMARY SLEEP DISORDERS

Treatments for sleep apnea, periodic limb movement disorder, and restless legs syndrome are dealt with in separate chapters in this volume. The treatment approach for the various medical causes of insomnia is, whenever possible, to treat the underlying medical problem. When insomnia is caused by somatic pain, analgesics may help with sleep by their inherent sedating qualities, as well as by diminishing the noxious stimuli that tend to awaken the patient or keep him awake.

5.1.6. LIGHT AND CIRCADIAN RHYTHMS

Variability in sleep-wake schedules may disrupt circadian physiology, leading to poor sleep. Research data in recent years has elucidated the critical role that light exposure plays in regulating circadian rhythms. Light exposure at specific times of the day helps to maintain and establish circadian rhythms. Since exposure to morning sunlight plays an important role in maintaining a stable and desired rhythm of sleep and wakefulness, a regular morning hour of arousal (and light exposure) is particularly important in maintaining a regular sleep rhythm. A regular hour of rising, as well as a regular bedtime, is beneficial in maintaining stable and strong sleep-wake patterns resulting from their capacities to recruit other circadian rhythms to the sleep-wake cycle.

5.1.7. CONCLUSIONS

Various treatment approaches for the psychophysiological insomnias have been suggested. For the transient or situational insomnias, if the initiating or inciting stress can be removed, the insomnia will likely disappear. If this is not possible, it is helpful for the involved clinician to take a supportive stance, emphasizing the acute and usually self-limited nature of the problem. Therapeutic strategies may include tactics such as regularization of the daily sleep and waking schedule, not spending time in bed if sleep remains elusive, not going to bed until tired, not remaining in bed if unable to sleep, and not using the bed or bedroom for nonsleep activities such as reading, eating, and watching television. Support by family members and friends should be encouraged.

Behavioral approaches to the treatment of persistent insomnias are discussed in detail in several of the references listed at the end of this chapter.

5.2. Pharmacologic Therapy of Insomnia

The general pharmacology of hypnotic/sedative use in sleep medicine is dealt with in Chapter 7. Although hypnotic agents are often used in the treatment of insomnia, a number of problems are associated with their use. For almost a century, physicians have expressed concern about the deleterious effects of hypnotic drugs. In recent years, it has even been suggested that hypnotics may do more harm than good for many insomnia patients. In response to caregiver and physician compassion for their insomnia, patients frequently receive prescriptions for benzodiazepine hypnotics and similar sedatives. It has been estimated that 30–48% of hypnotic prescriptions go to patients over 60 years of age, with the majority used on a long-term basis. This is of concern, since chronic use of hypnotics has been shown to increase the risk of falls, both in the hospital and in other environments.

The treatment of insomnia should always be multi-dimensional:

- Pharmacologic assistance is often necessary.
- Specific behavioral techniques must be suggested and employed.
- The patient must be educated to take the problem seriously, but must also be reassured so as not to provoke counter-productive worrying.
- Appropriate goals must be set and gradually advanced.
- Contributing conditions such as depression must be treated.

The recognition that substances such as alcohol and the opiates can promote sleep dates back to prehistory; herbal and other "natural" sleep treatments are described in a variety of ancient Greek and Egyptian texts. In modern times, the benzodiazepines and other compounds with benzodiazepine-agonist properties are prescribed. The benzodiazepines are remarkably safe overall with regard to respiratory suppression in overdosage. However, toxicity is greatly increased when these compounds are combined with other agents that may suppress respiration (i.e., ethanol). Thus, the year 1970 marks a watershed era in pharmacologic treatment of insomnia with the initial availability of flurazepam, the first of the benzodiazepine hypnotics. Flurazepam assumed a primary position among the hypnotics during the decade of the 1970s, largely supplanting the older compounds such as chloral hydrate, barbiturates, and barbiturate-like compounds. A second phase in the progression of insomnia treatment began in the later 1970s with the release of shorter half-life hypnotics, triazolam, and temazepam, which competed with and largely replaced flurazepam. The 1990s saw the development of a group of hypnotic agents that act at benzodiazepine (BZD) receptor sites in the brain, but that have a nonBZD chemical structure. Zolpidem, a compound with a short half-life of approximately 2.5 hours, was the first nonBZD agent approved for release in the United States. Zaleplon, with an even shorter half-life of 1 hour, has been submitted for approval to the Food and Drug Administration and may be available for clinical use in 1999. Both zolpidem and zaleplon appear to have a greater affinity for the BZD-1 receptor sub-type; this may lead to a lower likelihood of abuse potential and of side effects such as memory impairment and confusion seen with typical BZD hypnotic agents, which are not receptor-selective.

5.2.1. EFFICACY OF HYPNOTIC MEDICATIONS

The efficacy of hypnotic medications over short periods of use (up to four weeks) is well established in the scientific literature in general. Studies have looked at patient populations using medication for longer than the four week periods typical for research studies and that correspond to prescription practices encouraged by the Food and Drug Administration (FDA). Balter and Uhlenhuth examined the beneficial and adverse effects of hypnotics used for variable periods of time, up to a year in duration. Most of these users of prescription hypnotics attributed positive effects to their sleep medications, with infrequent adverse effects. Over-the-counter hypnotics were less effective and were more likely to produce negative effects. The untreated insomnia group was more symptomatic than any of the medication groups. In another study, Balter and Uhlenhuth examined concerns about short half-life benzodiazepine hypnotics from an epidemiologic perspective, drawing on survey data. In populations representative of outpatient practice, findings included a similar abuse liability for short compared to longer elimination half-life benzodiazepine hypnotics. Prevalence rates for serious accidents and injuries were much higher for chronic untreated insomnia than for normal controls and most other groups treated with psychotherapeutic medications. A high proportion of past users of hypnotics were satisfied with their medication and would take medications again if needed.

5.2.2. DRUG WITHDRAWAL INSOMNIA

Treatment of drug withdrawal insomnia and withdrawal states from alcohol or sedative drugs necessitates cautious gradual reduction in dose. Supervision of this process may require a period of treatment of from weeks to months.

5.2.3. REBOUND INSOMNIA

Rebound insomnia, defined as insomnia after discontinuation of medication that is worse than the pretreatment condition, is a problem seen with many hypnotic medications, particularly shorter-acting ones. It is characterized by a physical withdrawal syndrome, with general malaise as well as increases in anxiety and insomnia, occurring on discontinuation of treatment of from several weeks (usually) to as short as several days (rarely) duration. There are some data suggesting that rebound is less likely to be seen after discontinuation of zolpidem than other short half-life compounds such as triazolam.

5.2.4. SAFETY

All available sedative agents can produce dose- and concentration-dependent sedation, drowsiness, performance impairment, and amnesia. The presence of side effects with these compounds, consequently, should not be a source of surprise, and should be considered in deliberations regarding the use of these medications. However, all benzodiazepine and benzodiazepine-agonist compounds are remarkably safe in general use. The newer agents are safe in single agent overdose, although in combination with other drugs or alcohol, fatal results can occur.

5.2.5. GENERAL SIDE EFFECTS

The risk of carryover effects of long half-life agents has been a long-standing concern and has been demonstrated using the Multiple Sleep Latency Test and other performance and epidemiologic measures. Several studies have demonstrated increased risks for hip fracture in elderly patients using any class of compounds with long elimination half-lives—hypnotics, anxiolytics, tricyclic antidepressants, and antipsychotics—compared with the risks for individuals using short elimination half-life hypnotic-anxiolytics.

5.3. Antidepressants for Treatment of Insomnia

Antidepressant medications are used to treat insomnia in several contexts with separate rationales. First, of course, is the treatment of a major depression in which insomnia was a prominent symptom. Second, for patients being treated with newer antidepressants that may have "energizing" properties, especially the specific serotonin reuptake inhibitors (SSRIs), disruption of sleep and insomnia complaints are often reported, especially in the early phases of treatment. It has become common practice to use an agent with sedating properties to treat this drug-promoted insomnia complaint, either a benzodiazepine agonist such as zolpidem or temazepam, or a sedating antidepressant such as trazodone or doxepin. When antidepressants such as trazodone or doxepin are used, an additional rationale supporting their use is the supposition that the sleep-promoting antidepressant may have additive or synergistic effects in combination with the SSRI.

Finally, in patients with insomnia complaints independent of mood disturbance, sedating antidepressant compounds have long been used as primary hypnotics. Various rationales are cited to support this use. It is argued that the benzodiazepines and benzodiazepine agonist compounds are sometimes abused, lead to tolerance and habituation, and carry risks of problems such as rebound insomnia, daytime sedation, and disinhibition reactions. On such grounds, it can be argued that tricyclic and other antidepressants are rational alternatives to the primary hypnotic compounds. However, the tricyclic compounds have risks of their own, such as anticholinergic toxicity, orthostatic hypotension, and risk of falls, cardiotoxic effects, promotion of confusional states, and significant risk of death with overdosage.

Although the use of antidepressant medications in the treatment of insomnia complaints is widespread, there is remarkably little published supporting the safety and efficacy of this "off-label" (non–FDA approved or indicated for this condition) use of these medications. Among the antidepressants most often used as primary hypnotic agents are amitriptyline and doxepin, the tricyclic agents, and the heterocyclic agent trazodone. Doses used cover a broad range based on individual experience and preference but are often prescribed in a dosage range of 10–50 mg for amitriptyline and doxepin and 25–100 mg for trazodone. Limiting factors to the use of these agents are typical side effects seen with tricyclic agents, including complaints of constipation, dry mouth, urinary retention, and daytime sedation. Although anticholinergic side effects are seen less often with trazodone, similar complaints may be reported, as well as complaints of morning sedation and feelings of "fuzzy-headedness."

Are there advantages to these compounds as alternatives to benzodiazepines and benzodiazepine agonist compounds? Perhaps, but not necessarily. Certainly, diversion and abuse of the benzodiazepines is avoided by the use of antidepressants, but these are not problems frequently seen in many insomnia patient populations. For many patients in whom there is the hypothesis that depression plays a role in the presentation of insomnia, it may be hoped that the antidepressant, even if given in a presumably subtherapeutic dose, will provide some antidepressant benefit. Similarly, some patients may be receptive to receiving a medication in treatment of a "neurotransmitter disorder," which causes them to have disturbed mood and sleep who would otherwise refuse to take a medication.

6. SLEEP CONSULTATION AND SLEEP STUDIES FOR THE INSOMNIA PATIENT

The primary care practitioner should be able to treat effectively most patients with transient insomnia, and should feel comfortable prescribing hypnotic medications for at least a short-term treatment period (doses and regimens are given in Chapter 7). Most primary care practitioners should also be able to counsel the patient on sleep hygiene and stimulus control techniques. Educational handouts are helpful. Some practitioners and some patients may be comfortable with nightly use of hypnotic medications over a longer term, if there are no apparent negative consequences. Concerns about long-term use of hypnotic medications include tolerance, dose escalation, and neurocognitive deficits (most often seen in the elderly, in whom subtle changes may be missed).

Consultation with a sleep specialist can be helpful because:

- specific and detailed educational materials can be given to the patient;
- the patient might be reassured that his or her doctor is taking the complaint seriously;
- greater time for analysis can be devoted to finding the causes of the problem; and
- the appropriateness of additional testing can be determined.

The decision whether to refer for formal sleep consultation will depend on the specifics of each patient's condition and history. Referral may allow greater time to evaluate complicated aspects of insomnia, to assess possible excessive use of medication and to institute a plan for drug withdrawal, or to educate the patient in specific behavioral techniques.

Is there a role for sleep studies in the evaluation of the insomnia patient? Polysomnography (PSG) provides the capacity to obtain diagnostic information about many relevant physiological systems in sleep, including EEG, EKG, leg muscle activity, body movement, fine and gross motor behaviors (via video recording), respiration, blood oxygen and carbon dioxide levels, gastric pH, penile erections, and so forth. It is certainly true that data obtained from the PSG makes it much less likely that an occult source sleep disturbance of will be overlooked. However, in view of the considerable expense and inconvenience of laboratory sleep studies, as well as questions of the accuracy of a single night of testing in the insomniac patient, it is generally difficult to justify a PSG as part of the initial evaluation of the insomnia patient. The goal of the treating physician should be to establish a working diagnosis on the basis of the medical and sleep history and the physical examination and to delineate a treatment regimen based on the patient's specific findings and history. If this treatment approach is unsuccessful, and if specific treatment questions can be addressed in a sleep study that cannot be answered in other fashions (i.e., periodic limb movements in sleep in a patient without a bed partner; occult sleep apnea as a cause of midnocturnal awakenings) PSG may be helpful. It may also be appropriate to proceed with a sleep study if the agent proposed for treatment for a presumptive disorder may carry risks or raise concerns with regard to long-term use that would be minimized by study data establishing the presence of a specific disorder (i.e., clonazepam, opiates, or levodopa-carbidopa in treatment of periodic limb movements in sleep).

Other less involved sleep recording techniques may also be used, including unattended home PSG recording, home sleep studies with limited channels of recording, and sleep actigraphy. Each of these techniques provides substantially less data than attended laboratory recording, but may be of benefit as an alternative to the PSG or when polysomnography is not available.

CASE STUDIES

Case 1

Mrs. A., a 41-year-old divorced female, presented with a complaint of chronically disturbed sleep with nightly use of hypnotic medications for many years. The daughter of a physician, she remembered having been given "diet pills" as a teenager to control weight, hypnotics when sleep was elusive, and analgesics to control menstrual discomfort. Trained as a psychotherapist, she was distressed about her incapacity to sleep without medications but felt powerless to sleep without them. She did not feel sleepy at any fixed or regular bedtime hour, and relied on medications, usually clonazepam 2 mg, to "put her to sleep" on a regular nightly basis. Her sources of clonazepam were her primary physician and several physician friends, none of whom were aware that she was using this medication on a daily basis. She perceived herself to be obtaining as little as three hours of sleep per night, and reported feeling "fatigued and out of it mentally" in the daytime. However, she denied frank sleepiness, and reported an Epworth Scale score of 4 (normal).

Her home life was chaotic. She had full parental responsibility for her two daughters, ages 9 and 14. She had an irregular bedtime routine, often remaining up and active as late as 2 or 3 AM performing family chores (i.e., laundry, cleaning) or paperwork. On other nights, she would feel "exhausted physically, but not sleepy" and would get into bed as early as 9 PM to relax and try to fall asleep. She reported inability to fall asleep on any night without medication.

Her nine-year-old had difficulty falling asleep in her own room but would usually begin the night there before coming into her mother's room in the hours after midnight, reporting "bad dreams" that had awakened her. Mrs. A. reported that unless she allowed her daughter to sleep with her in her bed that the daughter would not be able to return to sleep. She acknowledged that it was "comforting" to have her daughter sharing her bed and also recognized that it was disruptive to her sleep to have to try to deal with her daughter's sleep complaints in the middle of the night.

She reported at least three awakenings per night, some caused by her daughter's sleep problems and some of unknown causation. She denied awareness of leg movement activity and denied restless leg complaints.

There was no history of snoring or observed apnea activity. When she awakened, she knew that she would not be able to return to sleep, and would then take an additional dose of clonazepam. She awakened (with difficulty) for child care responsibilities in the morning (i.e., preparing breakfasts and lunches), and would then return to bed at 8:30 AM for additional sleep after her children had left for school, on occasion taking another dose of clonazepam to facilitate this extra sleep. She reported awakening by 10:00 to 11:00 AM to begin her daytime activities. She reported obtaining very little natural light in the daytime, none in morning hours.

DIAGNOSES

1. Inadequate sleep hygiene.
2. Irregular sleep-wake pattern.
3. Delayed sleep phase syndrome.
4. Hypnotic-dependent sleep disorder.
5. Chronic psychophysiological insomnia.
6. Extrinsic sleep disorder not otherwise specified (daughter's sleep disturbance).
7. Dysthymia and anxiety symptoms, possibly secondary to or exacerbated by sleep disruption and deprivation.

DISCUSSION AND TREATMENT HISTORY

This case demonstrates the multifactorial nature of many insomnia disturbances. Elements of poor sleep conditioning, circadian rhythm disturbance, psychiatric disturbance, and chronic hypnotic use combine to create a condition of insomnia with multiple interacting components. It is difficult to identify all the contributory elements, but it is necessary if effective treatment is to be provided. In this case, treatment began by stabilizing the sleep environment and medication regimens. The patient was educated about the need to help her daughter overcome the sleep disturbance that she had developed (limit-setting disorder), and the patient's involvement in the process (in order to have company in her bed) was elucidated and explored. She was instructed to stabilize her night time routines and forbidden from engaging in mentally and physically stimulating activities after 9 PM. She was encouraged to increase her morning exposure to light, and instructed in basic elements of the stimulus control technique. Repeat doses of medication were forbidden during the night.

The patient called in panic after several days, reporting increases in awakening during the night, incapacity to set limits with her daughter, and a greater level of anxiety, depression, and fatigue during the daytime. She was encouraged to continue with the regimen, and allowed to increase her bedtime dose of clonazepam from 2 mg to 4 mg. At one week after initiation of her treatment program, she reported some improvement in her daughter's capacity to remain in her own bedroom through the night, and a greater sense of sleepiness at her desired bed-time hour of 11:30 PM. Anxious and depressive symptoms were present in the daytime, without other signs of benzodiazepine withdrawal. Trazodone 50 mg was added to the bedtime medication regimen, and the importance of morning sunlight as a part of her treatment regimen was emphasized to Mrs. A.

Over the next three weeks, the dose of trazodone was raised to 150 mg, and the clonazepam was reduced to 1 mg. Mrs. A's daughter became capable of falling asleep and remaining asleep within her own bedroom, a source of pride and satisfaction for her and her mother. Although Mrs. A. reported a continuing tendency for at least one awakening each night, she was better able to return to sleep and pleased that she had been able to reduce her use of clonazepam, particularly in view of her having used this without prescription or medical supervision. She reported that she was taking a morning walk two to three mornings per week. Mood was improved and more stable in the daytime, and she reported a greater sense of confidence about her capacity to re-establish a "normal" sleep pattern.

Six weeks after the initial visit, Mrs. A. reported that her sleep patterns had normalized to a degree that she had not experienced for at least fifteen years. She had increased morning activity and light exposure to at least five times per week, was falling asleep within twenty minutes of her bedtime, and sleeping through until the morning most nights. She had discontinued the clonazepam completely. She remained somewhat ambivalent about the continued use of trazodone, but she recognized that this was an important element, at least in the short term, in maintaining a stable and controlled sleep pattern. She agreed to continue to chart her sleep patterns and to return at monthly intervals, with a plan to decrease and/or discontinue trazodone within six months, if possible.

Although this was a complicated case which required detailed exploration of lifestyle and attitudes, the improvement was accomplished primarily by following routine sleep hygiene principles for both the patient and the family. The medication change was significant not so much in the change from one chemical class to another (benzodiazepine to antidepressant), but in the understanding of its proper role and use.

Case 2

Mrs. B., a 48-year-old female, presented for evaluation of complaints of difficulties initiating and maintaining sleep. Symptoms had been present for the preceding two years, but had increased in severity in the previous four months. She reported experiencing increased levels of anxiety during the daytime and evening hours, which she related to the challenges of her responsibilities as a self-employed small business person and reported that sleep was not fully restorative for her. She denied awareness of snoring or apneas, a finding confirmed by her husband. She denied complaints of excessive sleepiness even in sedentary settings, but she did confirm the presence of depressed mood, anhedonia, poor appetite and loss of 10 pounds, poor attention and concentration, a low energy level, and increasing feelings of anxiety and guilt.

Mrs. B. was reluctant to consider depression as the explanation for her sleep problems, but she did acknowledge having experienced problems with depression in the past. She reported one episode of postpartum depression at age 23, following the birth of her second child, and an episode that occurred "for no reason" about ten years prior to her sleep consultation. She confirmed a family history of affective illness, reporting that her mother and sister had both experienced repeated problems with depression. She acknowledged her tendencies to be a "controlling and strong-willed" individual and believed her incapacity to overcome her problems with sleep and depression reflected "moral and personal inadequacy." She recognized that some of her ambivalence regarding depression reflected her fears of becoming chronically depressed and disabled, as had her mother.

Mrs. B. expressed anxiety about her possibly becoming "addicted" to sleeping pills if she took them but was willing to try a low dose of a sedating antidepressant for sleep as an alternative to a benzodiazepine receptor agonist hypnotic.

DIAGNOSIS
1. Major depressive disorder.
2. Insomnia secondary to depression.

DISCUSSION AND TREATMENT HISTORY
Mrs. B. returned after three weeks of treatment, reporting little change in status overall, with the possible exception of some minor improvement in sleep. She agreed to an increase in dose of her antidepressant, and within several days of the increase in dose she began to note improvement in sleep, mood, energy level, and capacity for pleasure. Despite her concerns about "prolonged" use of any medication, she agreed to continue her use of the antidepressants for a period of at least four months in view of the substantial improvement that she had experienced. She maintained her degree of improvement during her six-

month period of treatment, but when medications were tapered, the discontinued symptoms of depression returned. Antidepressant treatment was resumed with good results, with the agreement to consider another effort at discontinuation of medication after an additional stable treatment period of six months.

Case 3

When seen in consultation, Mrs. C., a 56-year-old white female, the wife of a physician, was referred for evaluation of long-standing sleep complaints. She described her sleep complaint as follows:

With the help of medications I am able to sleep for two to four hours. When I wake up I am fully awake no matter what the hour.

Her sleep problems had been present for over 15 years. Severe problems with fibromyalgia had lead to a substantial decline in functioning. Amitriptyline, prescribed by her rheumatologist, had at one time been helpful for her in controlling pain and improving sleep but had been discontinued due to anticholinergic side effects. Other antidepressants that had been used singly or in combination in the past included doxepin and nortriptyline. She had received various sedative medications in treatment of sleep complaints, including clonazepam, triazolam, temazepam, chloral hydrate, meprobamate, ethchlorvynol, and various barbiturates. In reviewing her history of hypnotic use, it became apparent that she had in fact used hypnotic medications on a nightly basis for over 30 years.

She reported that she took her sleep medication, temazepam 30 mg, two to two-and-a-half hours before her regular hour of retiring of 11 PM. She awakened several hours later without awareness of any specific cause and reported difficulty in returning to sleep on a nightly basis. She listened to self-help and relaxation tapes on a nightly basis, keeping the recorder running throughout the night whether she was awake or asleep.

She reported that she "rested" for an hour at a time several times a day, denying true sleepiness but acknowledging symptoms of fatigue and low energy. "On rare occasions" she could recognize that she had fallen asleep briefly during these periods of daytime "rest."

Diagnosis
1. Chronic psychophysiological insomnia.
2. Hypnotic-dependent sleep disorder.
3. Sleep-state misperception.

Discussion and Treatment History

Treatment was initiated to reduce reliance on medications, to improve sleep hygiene, to increase her recognition about the amount of sleep she was actually obtaining, and to improve nocturnal sleep continuity. A modified stimulus control approach was used. She was restricted to a single 20-minute period of rest or sleep in the afternoon. Use of her tape recorder during the night was forbidden, and her sleep medication was changed to zolpidem to allow for more rapid onset of action and shorter duration of action. She was told to not go to bed until she felt tired in the evening, and to take her sleep medication at that time. She was instructed to avoid clock-watching during the night, and if she awakened during the night and could not return to sleep, she was told to get up from bed and read something relaxing or boring in another room until she felt sleepy, at which point she could return to bed. She was asked to complete a sleep diary on a daily basis.

Her initial perception was that she was obtaining somewhat less sleep than had previously been her norm, with a further decline in daytime performance. Over a period of four weeks, her reported sleep time in bed at night climbed to five hours, with improvement in perceived daytime function. Over the next year, with monthly visits to provide support during behavioral interventions and implementation of good sleep hygiene, she was able to taper and discontinue routine use of zolpidem, reporting a substantial improvement in her fibromyalgia symptoms and her sleep complaints. She would use zolpidem "as needed" for stress and flare-ups in her fibromyalgia, on average less than three times per month.

Over a period of five years, sleep complaints and fibromyalgia symptoms have waxed and waned, usually in association with levels of stress. She has resumed regular use of zolpidem during periods of stress, but continues to effectively use behavioral techniques to avoid a nightly pattern of use.

SUGGESTED READINGS

Ancoli-Israel S. *All I Want Is A Good Night's Sleep*. Mosby-Year Book, St. Louis, 1996.

Consensus Development Conference. Drugs and insomnia: the use of medication to promote sleep. *JAMA* 1984; 251: 2410–2414.

Diagnostic Classification Steering Committee, Thorpy, M., Chairman. *ICSD-International classification of sleep disorders: diagnostic and coding manual*. American Sleep Disorders Association, Rochester, MN, 1990.

Balter M, Uhlenhuth E. The beneficial and adverse effects of hypnotics. *J Clin Psych* 1991; 52 Suppl: 16–23.

Erman M (ed). *Sleep Disorders. The Psychiatric Clinics of North America*, Vol 10, No 4, December. W.B. Saunders Company, Philadelphia, 1997.

Hauri P, Linde S. *No More Sleepless Nights*, John Wiley & Sons, New York City, 1990.

Hauri P. (ed). *Case Studies in Insomnia*, Plenum Publishing, New York City, 1991.

Kupfer D, Reynolds C. Current concepts: management of insomnia. *N Engl J Med* 1997; 336: 341–346.

Morin C. *Insomnia: Psychological Assessment and Management*, Guilford Press, New York City, 1993.

3

The Uses of Bright Light in an Office Practice

How to Brighten Up Your Patients

Daniel F. Kripke

CONTENTS

1. CIRCADIAN RHYTHMS AND LIGHT

Fresh air, exercise, and a healthy diet have been the nostrums of physicians throughout history. Modern physicians have been forgetting the "fresh air," which we can now understand as the value of outdoor daylight. A more scientific understanding of the value of daylight has developed recently. Moreover, we have learned how a physician can substitute bright artificial light to help patients who no longer spend much time outdoors.

1.1. Many Patients Experience Little Light

My colleagues and I have measured how much time people spend outdoors in a random population sample of middle-aged adults in San Diego. Our measurements show that in San Diego, California, people are outdoors in daylight less than one hour per day on average. Although some people are outdoors for hours, shopping, playing golf, or strolling

From: *Sleep Disorders: Diagnosis and Treatment*
Edited by: J. S. Poceta and M. M. Mitler © Humana Press Inc., Totowa, NJ

Table 1
Approximate Illumination of Human Environments

Environment	Lux[a]	Foot candle
Starlight	0.01	0.001
Full moon	1	0.1
Office (looking toward the desk or wall)	50–500	5–50
Rainy or cloudy day outdoors	500–2000	50–200
Full sunlight at noon	10,000	1000

[a]One lux is the illumination given by one candle at 1 meter from a surface. One foot candle is the illumination given by one candle at one foot from a surface. Therefore, one foot candle is 10.76 lux.

on the beach, a larger number stay indoors almost all day and never spend substantial time in daylight. Although the finding of a low average daylight exposure is important, the range of exposures is even more impressive. In the course of a day, some adults are exposed to one thousand times as many photons as their more dismal neighbors. Of course, San Diego is one of the most pleasant coastal cities in Southern California. We have more sunshine than 82% of American cities. Moreover, in San Diego, it is rarely too hot or too cold to go outdoors. Phoenix has more sunshine than San Diego, but it is often too hot to be outdoors in the summer. Similarly, many cities have generous sunshine in the winter, but are very cold.

With colleagues at the Mayo Clinic in Rochester, Minnesota, we compared people's light exposures in San Diego with the pattern in Rochester. In the summer, people in Rochester were out in daylight a bit more than in San Diego, perhaps because summer days are longer further north, or perhaps because farming is more prevalent in Minnesota. In winter, on the other hand, people in Rochester were in daylight only about 20% as much as people in San Diego, owing primarily to the temperature differential. Moreover, in larger cities, people might see even less winter daylight than in Rochester, because many cities are now built for traveling underground. For example, in Toronto a person can take the subway to work and walk for blocks underground to arrive at the office or shopping center without ever setting foot outside.

People think they have plenty of lighting indoors. This perception is often quite deceptive, because visual needs and photobiologic needs are quite different. The human eye has an ability to adjust to an astonishing range of lighting without our being aware. We can see throughout a visual range of more than six orders of magnitude (2×10^6) or 2 million-fold, from 0.01 lux to about 20,000 lux (Table 1). Although illumination

Light affects the brain and the sleep-wake cycle because:

- The light stimulates receptors in the retina.
- The retino-hypothalamic tract reaches the suprachiasmatic nucleus and other hypothalamic nuclei.
- Sympathetic fibers descend into the superior cervical ganglion, and then ascend to the pineal gland.
- In the pineal, serotonin is converted to melatonin.
- Melatonin has cellular effects including feedback to the suprachiasmatic nucleus.

may exceed 100,000 lux at noon looking at the sun, we obviously never look directly at the noontime sun. On a sunny day, illumination may be about 10,000 lux looking towards the horizon. Indoors, people spend most of their time in environments lit at less than 100 lux in the direction of gaze. In the evening, the average living room might be lit at about 15 lux, but some people watch television in rooms as dim as 1 lux, which is about the same as the light of the full moon.

1.2. The Body Clock and Phase Resetting

We really do have a 24-hour clock inside our bodies in the suprachiasmatic nucleus, a hypothalamic area just above the optic chiasm. The individual neurons of the suprachiasmatic nucleus (SCN) are capable of developing rhythms of about 24 hours, which we call *circadian* ("about a day") rhythms. As a whole, the neurons of the SCN constitute a circadian pacemaker or timing mechanism for the body. The suprachiasmatic nucleus receives neural impulses from the eye through the optic nerves. Basically, bright light influences the SCN to keep our body clocks on schedule. The SCN controls the pineal gland through a multisynaptic pathway that includes the paraventricular nucleus of the hypothalamus, descending fibers to the spinal cord, the preganglionic sympathetic fibers, which reach the superior cervical ganglion in the neck, and the postganglionic sympathetic fibers that climb next to the carotid artery and its branches to reach the pineal.

The effect of sympathetic norepinephrine on the pineal gland is to cause the serotonin (manufactured from tryptophan in the pineal) to be converted to melatonin. Melatonin is a highly lipid-soluble hormone that rapidly diffuses into the circulation and reaches every cell in the body. Melatonin seems to have two effects on the hypothalamus: it feeds back on the phase timing of the SCN, and it controls hormones such as the pituitary gonadotropins. For example, in Siberian hamsters, melatonin makes the testicles and ovaries atrophy and the hair turn white—an interesting fact that I feel my patients should know!

Melatonin is a night hormone which is elevated at night in both diurnal and nocturnal animals (1). Light suppresses pineal production of melatonin. Some researchers suspect that melatonin triggers the onset of sleepiness in humans, but melatonin could not be a simple sleep-inducing hormone, since high melatonin is accompanied by higher alertness in nocturnal animals. Moreover, pinealectomized animals that synthesize almost no melatonin seem to sleep reasonably well. Whether melatonin is important in triggering sleep in humans, or whether melatonin is just a marker of SCN timing remains controversial. Similarly, the endocrine effects of melatonin in humans remain little understood, such as antigonadal effects.

Our body clocks can run slightly fast or slow just as mechanical watches do. Thousands of years ago, when humans were still sleeping outside, the light of dawn probably set the SCN each morning, somewhat like great grandfather used to set his pocket watch every morning by the time broadcast on the radio. The tendency for our body clocks to run fast or slow, and the way in which the timing is affected by light, underpin our understanding of the circadian rhythm disorders.

For animals and plants that spend their lives outdoors, light affects the body clock according to a "phase-response curve" that is basically similar for most organisms. The sensitive phase of the phase response curve normally occurs at night when there is little light. Evening light tends to delay the body clock, so that sleep onset, melatonin secretion, and other parameters occur somewhat later. Were the body clock too fast so that it drifted early, the sunlight before dusk would hit that part of the phase-response curve that delays rhythms, and the timing would tend to be corrected. Conversely, somewhat after the normal midsleep time (for example, after about 3–5 AM among people sleeping from 11 PM to 6 AM), there is an advance portion of the phase response mechanism. Morning light, especially from about 6–10 AM, may cause sleep onset, morning awakening, the end of nocturnal melatonin secretion, and other functions to commence earlier. The morning portion of the phase-response curve would correct any body clock tendency to drift too late. The basic functional properties of the human phase-response curve are important, because they can guide us clinically to treat common patient complaints.

2. ADVANCED AND DELAYED SLEEP-PHASE SYNDROMES

Our human body clocks do sometimes seem to run too fast or too slow, or at least the timing drifts too early or too late, so that circadian

The phase response curve is an experimentally determined construct that predicts the effect of light on circadian rhythms.

- Bright light administered in the morning tends to advance circadian rhythms (move them earlier in the subsequent cycle).
- Bright light administered in the evening tends to delay circadian rhythms.
- The portions of the day which are most predictable and most sensitive to these effects tend to be the hours near the bedtime and wake-up time.

rhythms become relatively advanced or delayed. In modern society, for people who are not outdoors much so that the sun can adequately set the circadian pacemaker, two distinct problems can occur. These body clock problems are associated with advance or delay of the circadian phase.

2.1. Advanced Sleep-Phase

When the body clock becomes advanced, functions controlled by the body clock occur too early. Usually, sleep symptoms are the most important signs of what we call "advanced sleep-phase syndrome." The chief symptoms of advanced sleep-phase are falling asleep too early and waking up too early. People with an advanced sleep-phase typically nod off in the evening reading or watching television. They may fall asleep before they retire to bed, even needing to be awakened to go to bed and turn off the lights. A more dangerous problem would be falling asleep behind the wheel of a car in the evening. Likewise, the person with advanced sleep-phase awakens too early. This patient's internal rhythm may awaken him or her at 3 AM, 4 AM, or 5 AM, long before the rooster crows. Patients are distressed when they would like to sleep later, even though patients with advanced sleep-phase often feel most energetic in the morning. Also, if the people with advanced sleep-phase somehow manages to stay up to a customary bedtime, they will usually still wake up early, thus producing insufficient time for sleep, sleep deprivation, and sleepiness the next day.

Some experts have questioned whether advanced sleep-phase syndrome truly ever occurs. If one defines the "syndrome" in a very extreme way, it may be quite rare, but it would be nonsense to deny that many patients are troubled by falling asleep too early and by awakening too early. Indeed, past 40 years of age, complaints of awakening too early seem to be more common than complaints of trouble falling sleep.

Advanced sleep-phase might be partly a social condition. A hundred and fifty years ago, when most people lived on farms, and there was little artificial lighting besides candles, it may have been customary to fall asleep at 8 or 9 PM and awaken at 4 or 5 AM to tend the farm at dawn. Incidentally, the lifestyle of farm animals is in synchronicity with the natural light cycle, so that many animals get half of their sleep before midnight and spend half of their waking hours before noon. In a pre-21st century society, it has become customary to stay up after dark for social activities or prime time television. Often, people do not start working before 9 AM. In this social context, the normal sleep patterns of one hundred fifty years ago may now be perceived as a sleep disorder. Advanced sleep-phase may be partly an incompatibility of natural biology with the latest social customs.

Advanced sleep-phase seems to be much more common in the elderly. One theory for which there is some laboratory evidence is that our body clocks speed up as we age, even though most body processes slow down. A faster body clock would continue to run slightly fast unless repeatedly reset. Deterioration of vision may also be a factor in causing advanced-sleep-phase tendencies to be more common in the elderly as compared to the young. As the lenses of our eyes become cloudy and opacify into cataracts, elders see "as through a glass, darkly," so that much less light strikes the retina. With the eyes' remarkable ability to adapt to changes in lighting, patients may not recognize clouding of the lenses until almost 99% of the light falling on the corneas has been obscured. Older people also have smaller pupils, which further decreases the light reaching the retina. Finally, macular degeneration and other retinal problems may impair the eyes' light-sensing mechanisms. All of these eye problems might cause elderly people to need extra light to make a normal adjustment of the body clock (2). Advanced sleep-phase also seems to be more common among elderly women compared to men. We do not know why, but several studies have shown that among people of retirement age, the daily rhythms of women are set, on average, about an hour earlier. This might be a factor that makes insomnia more common among elderly women, as it is a fact that after menopause, women complain of insomnia much more than men do.

As previously mentioned, advanced sleep-phase might be partly a social mismatch of our bodies' biology and modern society, but adequate light exposure would probably minimize this mismatch. The great enemy of good lighting seems to be television. People watch more and more television or computer screens, which often are equally dim. A wedding of televisions, computers, and telephones may be on the way, in which life may become centered on the screens. Because television screens are really not very bright, many people watch them in rather dark rooms. In actual measurements of people from 60–79 years of age, we have found that the average evening lighting is quite dim. Perhaps 10% are spending the evening (most likely watching television) in 1 lux or less! It is not hard to understand that the dim lighting of some TV rooms and living rooms is insufficient to make the body clock react as if it were still day and still the time to remain awake. A second enemy of good lighting is energy conservation. Although the principle of conserving electricity is worthy, turning off the lights too zealously can cause real medical illness for trivial savings.

2.2. Treatment of Advanced Sleep-Phase Syndrome

Solving advanced sleep-phase is very simple for many people. Often, all that is needed is a brighter lamp by the television chair. I have found that 300-watt lamps are often sufficient. Halogen-bulb "torchiere" lamps which bounce light indirectly off of the ceiling may be particularly aesthetically acceptable and easy to install. There is no special advantage to these halogen lamps, except that they are inexpensive and easily accepted. The halogen bulb's very bright point of light and ultraviolet content might make it risky to look at a halogen bulb directly. Looking directly at a halogen bulb is never recommended. This is why the 300-watt halogen lamps are generally designed as indirect lighting. In fact, halogen lamps are inefficient because the light has to be bounced off the ceiling, whereas fluorescents with diffusers viewed directly are much more efficient. Electronic ballasts may reduce eye strain and headache related to fluorescents. Fluorescent light boxes can produce 10 to 30 times the lux measurement at the eye as a halogen lamp of similar wattage bouncing off the ceiling, which might produce only 200–300 lux. Nevertheless, 200–300 lux may be 10 to 100 times the previous lighting in a living room, and for many patients, this level of illumination would be sufficient.

For advanced sleep-phase, bright light should be used for 1–3 hours at a convenient point in the evening, often when a person is sitting in a chair reading or watching television. For some, obtaining bright light during dinner may be appropriate. It makes little difference if a person gets up and down from the chair near the light, as long as the person is in bright light most of the time. If a person does not stay in one room most of the evening, it may be necessary to brighten more than one room. Some people need a longer exposure than others, depending both on the brightness of the lighting and on individual factors. The later the bright light is used, the more powerful will be its effect. However, many people will find that they should dim down the lighting for about an hour

Table 2
Phase Symptoms and Treatments

Advanced sleep-phase	Delayed sleep-phase
Symptoms	Symptoms
Falling asleep too early in the evening	Trouble falling asleep or very late bedtime
Awakening too early in the morning	Trouble getting up in the morning or sleeping late
Treatments	Treatments
Treat with bright light in the evening	Treat with bright light in the morning
Use sun glasses outdoors before noon	Never oversleep, even on weekends

before they wish to go to bed, to avoid "overdosing" and causing trouble with falling asleep.

A person with advanced sleep-phase might begin to feel some benefit after using brighter evening light every night for a week, but it might take a month or two before the maximum benefit is reached, especially because it takes some time to restore good sleep habits. Once the problem is under control, and the body clock has readjusted, a person with advanced sleep-phase can often afford to skip bright evening light on special evenings when they wish to entertain or go out. Nevertheless, usage of brighter light in the evening probably needs to become a life-long habit, coupled with other good sleep habits. A person who benefits from bright evening light will often relapse within a month after skipping the bright light too often.

People with advanced sleep-phase should avoid very bright light very early in the morning, because morning light would further advance a body clock which is already too advanced. Sometimes, outdoor exercise soon after dawn or a long drive to work in the morning contributes to the problem. A person with advanced sleep-phase can be advised to wear dark wrap-around sunglasses when outdoors between dawn and noon. Table 2 summarizes some of these concepts for the treatment of phase-shift disorders.

2.3. Advanced Sleep-Phase and Depression

There are indeed two conditions which typically cause early awakening: advanced sleep-phase and depression. There seems to be some relationship between advanced sleep-phase and depression, particularly in middle age and beyond. It may be difficult to distinguish the two conditions, but it is necessary to evaluate the severity of ancillary symptoms of depression. Bright light in the evening seems to work both for advanced sleep-phase and for depression with early awakening *(see Subheading 3)*, so sometimes it may not be important to distinguish which condition is most active in the patient.

2.4. Delayed Sleep-Phase

When the body clock runs too slow, it sends its various effector signals to the body too late—the phase of the body clock is delayed later than it should be. The symptoms of delayed sleep-phase are falling asleep too late, often after lying in bed for many hours, and waking up too late or having trouble getting up on time. People with delayed sleep-phase typically have trouble falling asleep unless they stay up much later than they would wish to. Having gone to sleep so late, people with delayed sleep-phase often oversleep and have trouble getting to work or carrying out morning activities, as if their bodies' internal alarm clocks do not ring on time. Indeed, people with severe delayed sleep-phase will sometimes sleep past noon. People with delayed sleep-phase—unless they drag themselves out of bed—are often rather long sleepers. They often feel somewhat rebellious or angry with authorities, perhaps because they have experienced so many years of people insisting that they wake up even though their body clocks are telling them to keep on sleeping. Unfortunately, people who do not come to school or work on time are often regarded as lazy or undependable. Also, since people with delayed sleep-phase may not feel alert until well past noon, and their best and most energetic hours are sometimes past midnight, they may have learned to enjoy their habitual late activities and may be reluctant to give them up for bed. All of these factors tend to solidify the rhythm at a later-than-desired time.

The timing of sleep patterns—advanced or delayed—seems to run in families. It is possible that people with delayed sleep-phase have a genetic change in the body clock. It is also peculiar that delayed sleep-phase seems to develop somewhat late in puberty— around 16 to 18 years of age—and the condition is often at its worst in the early 20's. College students and graduate students without fixed classes seem to be particularly prone to delayed sleep-phase. There is little quiet in the dormitories before midnight at our university. One wonders if that rebellious trait— the wish to get out from under the thumb of authority—sometimes enters into a delayed sleep-phase. There is even some evidence in animal studies that the younger adult animals adopt a different daily rhythm, apparently to keep out of the way of the more dominant more mature adults. Nevertheless, we do see delayed sleep-phase among mature adults and even in some elderly people as well as in young adults.

It is apparent that low light exposure has something to do with the development of delayed sleep-phase. We all get up later in winter—on standard time—than we do in the summer, when daylight savings time causes us to set our alarm clocks an hour earlier. Of course, the dawn is earlier in the summer as well. A number of studies indicate that even after taking account of the time change, people tend to stay up later and get up later in winter than in summer. This trend seems to be especially prominent in northern areas (above 45° latitude), where winter nights are particularly long. In those areas, people may see no bright daylight in the morning, because they arrive at school or work before the sun comes up. Theorists have speculated that experiencing dawn is particularly important for setting body clocks and even that the gradually waxing light of dawn has some special signaling significance for the body clock. Indeed, Stephanie Rosen in my laboratory found some evidence that people who have lighter window shades, which let in more dawn light, tend to fall asleep a little more rapidly and rise a little earlier *(3)*. Whether or not the waxing light of dawn is an important signal, it is clear that people whose sleep-phase is delayed are not experiencing sufficient bright light in the morning. This is the key to treatment.

2.5. Treatment of Delayed Sleep-Phase Syndrome

The best treatment for delayed sleep-phase is to increase the dose of light which the patient receives in the morning. The brighter the light, the sooner after waking up it is experienced, and the longer the period of exposure (up to three or four hours), the better the response is likely to be. Delayed sleep-phase is often a stubborn condition which can only be controlled by very bright light for one to two hours each morning. Arranging to receive that light may be hard to fit in with daily habits. There are many ways of arranging to get a little more bright light in the morning, such as installing bright lighting in the bathtub or around the bathroom mirror (i.e., dressing-room lights), increasing lighting in the bedroom and kitchen, and removing sunglasses when driving or walking to work. Although halogen torchiere lamps and other increased conventional lighting might sometimes be helpful, most indoor lighting does not seem to be sufficient for this condition. Sitting near a window or open curtains is rarely bright enough. Delayed sleep-phase usually requires a bright fluorescent light box. One convenient way to get a strong dose of morning light is to use such a bright light box (e.g., a box arranged for 10,000 lux) for 30 minutes at breakfast time, since eating and reading the morning paper do not interfere with the benefit. For people who work at a desk, placing the light box on the desk and turning it on all morning should be effective, even if one does not sit at the desk all of the morning. If it is convenient to be exposed to bright light for several hours each morning, around 2000 lux might well be sufficient, allowing the light box to be placed at the far side of the desk. The brightness of the light that reaches the retina is influenced by the exact position of the light and the eyes. Also, a higher (brighter) dose can achieve the same effect in a shorter time than a lesser dose over a longer time.

The exact timing of the light in the morning may be a bit complicated, since at the beginning, the patient's natural waking time may be quite late in the day. It is probably best to start using the bright light after the usual waking time, and then to move the treatment earlier and earlier in the day as the person starts falling asleep earlier and waking up earlier. If the weather permits, a rapid initial response can be achieved if the patient will go outdoors from about 8 AM until noon for the first two to three days. Once a person is able to fall asleep at a reasonable hour and to awaken at the desired time (e.g., 7 AM), the best time for treatment is soon after awakening in the early morning. In the first week or two of correcting delayed sleep-phase, it is very important to use bright light treatment for a full dose every day, seven days per week.

Just as it is harder to set an alarm clock for a new time than it is just to turn on the alarm once the time has been set, similarly, it takes less bright light to keep the body clock set properly after a delayed body clock has been reset. After a delayed body clock has been successfully readjusted, and the person's habits have also readjusted to the new sleep hours, a bit less effort may be needed to keep the body clock from delaying again. Nevertheless, people with delayed sleep-phase usually relapse if they stop using light treatment loyally. Also, it is very bad for patients with delayed sleep-phase to stay up late on Friday nights and to sleep late on weekends and days off. Their body clock will desire to shift later anytime it is allowed to do so. A person with delayed sleep-phase should try to keep a regular wake-up time, seven days per week, because once a little relapse is permitted on days off, the person with delayed sleep-phase will find it very difficult to recover. Table 2 summarizes some of these concepts for the treatment of phase shift disorders.

The theoretical importance of the dawn signal has inspired some doctors to try "dawn simulators," which slowly increase artificial room lighting in about the same pattern that dawn might creep through a bedroom window. Some believe that the natural dawn signal is so powerful that it will reset the body clock even during sleep, when the light has to pass through the eyelids, and that dawn simulation does not have to be very bright. Several dawn simulators designed to mimic the light of dawn are now being sold, although they have not been tested very well. There is preliminary evidence that dawn simulators have some benefit but not as powerful a benefit as a 10,000 lux light box *(4)*. Hopefully, dawn simulators will be more thoroughly tested, since they may be a particularly convenient way of dealing with delayed sleep-phase.

2.6. Depression and Delayed Sleep-Phase

Depression is occasionally associated with delayed sleep-phase, particularly among young adults and women before menopause, and particularly when the problem occurs in the winter (*see* Subheading 3). With delayed sleep-phase (as with advanced sleep-phase, as previously discussed), it is often difficult to tell when the problem is a sleep-timing problem and when it is a real depression, because they often are mixed together. Bright light which corrects delayed sleep-phase seems to lift mood symptoms as well.

3. BRIGHT LIGHT TREATMENT AND DEPRESSION

3.1. Depressions that Respond to Bright Light

A major depression can be diagnosed when a person feels depressed, down, sad, or gloomy most of the day nearly every day, or loses interest in normal pleasures. Moreover, by definition (for a depression to be "major"), the person with major depression has at least three or four additional symptoms such as weight loss or weight gain, loss of sleep (or sleeping too much), becoming agitated or slowed down, becoming fatigued, feeling guilty and worthless, losing the ability to concentrate, and actually thinking about death or suicide. When the condition is not so severe, it may be called a minor depression.

Sometimes a person experiences depression mainly in the winter—a pattern that seems to occur most commonly among women before the menopause. This pattern of winter seasonal trend in depression has been called "Seasonal Affective Disorder" (SAD). Unlike most depressions, people with SAD often say that they sleep in excess of their usual sleep, although it is sometimes more a matter of feeling fatigued and spending extra time in bed, rather than actually being asleep. Unlike the more common forms of depression, SAD patients often have a somewhat delayed sleep-phase and have particular problems in getting up in the morning. Among older patients with nonseasonal depressions, waking up early is more typical, but early awakening can occur in SAD also. Many people with seasonal affective disorder experience increased carbohydrate craving such as eating sweets, and they sometimes gain weight and need larger clothing in the winter, although loss of appetite can also occur in SAD. Some people with SAD feel withdrawn and want to curl up like a hibernating bear, but they may have fewer symptoms of

To conclude that a major depression is seasonal, certain criteria should be met:

- There has been a regular temporal relationship between the onset of the depression and a particular time of the year (usually fall or winter). Do not include cases in which there is an obvious effect of seasonal-related psychosocial stressors (e.g., regularly being unemployed every winter).
- Full remissions occur at a characteristic time of the year (e.g., depression disappears in the spring).
- In the last two years, two major depressive episodes have occurred that demonstrate the temporal seasonal relationships, and no nonseasonal episodes occurred during the same period.
- Seasonal depressive episodes substantially outnumber the nonseasonal depressive episodes that may have occurred over the individual's lifetime.

(Adapted from DSM-IV, American Psychiatric Association, 1994)

sadness and guilt than other major depressives. There is a milder form of SAD called subsyndromal SAD, which is simply more common, but less severe. People with the milder seasonal disorder suffer mild lethargy, gloom, and weight gain in the winter, sometimes oversleeping in the mornings, but not a really disabling depression.

It seems quite clear that many people with SAD have the winter pattern of recurrence at one time in their lives and the more common nonseasonal pattern on other occasions. In my opinion, both seasonal and nonseasonal depressions are probably somewhat different manifestations of the same illness. Some people have just one depression in a lifetime, but probably for most people with depression, this state is at least occasionally recurrent. The pattern of recurrence is extremely unpredictable for most people with depression, and most major depressions do not occur in the winter. Actually, depression is more commonly recognized in the spring, and occasionally in the fall, than either in winter or in summer.

Depressions occur more often in people who do not experience enough bright light. We have now studied more than 300 randomly selected people in San Diego who volunteered to wear an instrument for measuring how much light people experience. The trend was for people who experienced less bright lighting (largely because they spent less time in daylight) to report more depression. In San Diego, there is only a small difference in available daylight between summer and winter; consequently, the relationship of low light to depression could not be explained by the winter season. On the other hand, winter depression becomes increasingly common as one examines the more northern areas of the United States, especially Fairbanks and northern Alaska. It is very clear that as one moves north—and arrives at places with shorter, darker winter days—the prevalence of winter depression increases. Cold winter temperatures are also related to winter depression, which may suggest that part of winter depression is caused by cold weather keeping people indoors. As might be expected, the pattern of recurrent summer depression seems to be most common in the hottest parts of the US, although it does not seem as common as winter depression. It may be that summer temperatures that keep people indoors in air-conditioning (and out of daylight) are the explanation for this condition.

There is evidence that patients with major depressions benefit from treatment with bright light, whether or not the depression has a seasonal pattern. Relatively mild depressions—perhaps some not really meeting the criteria for "major" depression may also respond. Not surprisingly, there is some evidence that patients with more chronic and refractory depressions respond more poorly than those who have been down for only a matter of months, but neither chronicity nor lack of seasonal pattern is a contraindication to light treatment.

3.2. Using Bright Light Treatment for Depression

As a general rule, the more bright light that depressed patients receive, the more likely they are to begin feeling better. People vary in how much bright light they need to combat depressive symptoms. There must be many factors, including the severity of the depression. A more severe problem may need much more lighting to overcome depression. The amounts of light needed are somewhere in the range required to bring a depressed person above the average for daily light exposure. This can be achieved with as little as 15 to 30 minutes of very bright light (approaching 10,000 lux) or with a few hours of light of 2000–3000 lux (like a cloudy day in the shade). I would worry about the safety of choosing any brightness above about 10,000 lux, and I never recommend anything brighter. If the amount of depression is substantial, light much dimmer than 2000 lux is not likely to be effective without using many hours of daily exposure, although modest amounts of lighting may be sufficient for mild depression accompanying advanced sleep-phase in the elderly. The information now available about the effectiveness of different dosages is quite fragmentary. Moreover, we

---

The bright light treatment of depression is relevant to clinicians because:

• Light can be a useful addition to counselling and antidepressants.
• There is a marked association of insomnia with depression.
• Many patients have some combination of a circadian disorder, mood disorder, and sleep disorder.

---

suspect that in most studies, the planned dosages and the actual dosages received may not have corresponded very accurately. Thus, for the present time, somebody who wants to use bright light can only try and see how much light is needed.

The decision about whether to try 10,000 lux for a shorter time or 2000–3000 lux for a couple of hours depends on several things. Most people seem to prefer the brighter light for the shorter time because of the convenience of shortening the time required. Using 10,000 lux generally requires getting closer to the light source, which may be awkward in some settings. A full 10,000 lux will also make some people's eyes uncomfortable. Theoretically, we would expect 2000 lux to be safer for the eyes than 10,000 lux, but 10,000 lux has been tested enough now without any proof of eye damage that most experts seem quite confident of its safety. After all, 10,000 is no brighter than what we normally experience when we spend time outdoors on a bright day, and people have been testing that for longer than recorded history.

Like many other treatments, the timing and dosage of bright light needs to be individualized. It usually takes at least a week of using light every day to see some benefit, and there is often continuing improvement for at least a month of using a given dose of bright light. One should not get disappointed too quickly, especially if even slow improvement is noticeable. It is possible to use too much bright light. Eyestrain, headache, irritability, or sleep trouble may be some signs of excessive treatment.

For many patients, bright light at any time of day helps depression. Some studies comparing morning, afternoon, and evening bright light treatments show about equal results at various times of day. There is some evidence that many SAD patients may do a bit better with morning light (not every study agrees), but that may be not because of the seasonality of the depression but rather, because SAD patients tend to sleep late. Possibly, it is the sleep pattern that provides the most useful clue to optimal timing.

Using sleep symptoms to time light treatment is simple and follows the same principles as outlined for the circadian phase shift disorders. If a patient has trouble falling asleep and has trouble getting up on time each morning and thus seems phase-delayed, that person is likely to be most effectively treated using bright light early in the morning. People whose depression is linked to hypersomnia may also tend generally to do best with light in the morning. For such patients, the hour immediately after awakening is the most effective time to use bright light. In contrast, evening bright light is best for the patient who nods off early in the evening, who cannot stay awake for prime time television, and who awakens too early in the morning. For the person who does not fit clearly into either of these patterns, there might be little difference between morning and evening bright light treatment, and midday or afternoon bright light might work well also.

3.3. Duration of Bright Light Treatment

Many people who benefit from bright light need to use bright light for years. If they discontinue using light, after a few weeks, they may relapse into depression again. Some people find that they need less time with their light box to avoid relapse than they did to make the depression go away at the beginning. Therefore, after at least two to three months of remission, it could be reasonable to try slowly reducing the light dosage, to see if symptoms recur. Reducing the dosage is unlikely to be successful if progress is incomplete, because then relapse is more likely. The exception may be people with winter depression who have learned that their symptoms stop at a certain time of year, but experience often teaches even winter depressives to use light year round.

3.4. Combining Bright Light, Antidepressant Drugs, and Counseling

Bright light treatment should generally be combined with antidepressant drugs when treating serious depressions. For nonseasonal depressions, evidence suggests that the benefits from light treatment may be as great or greater in patients also receiving antidepressant drugs as compared to drug-free patients. There may be some synergy between light and pharmacotherapy, and certainly, there is no incompatibility. Although bright light was initially conceived as an alternative to pharmacotherapy for SAD, long-term data indicate that these treatments should often be combined (5). Combinations of bright light and psychotherapies have not been studied specifically, but there is no reason to doubt that combined treatment would be helpful.

Table 3
Using Light for Jet Lag

Flying east to west	*Flying west to east*
Before flying	Before flying
Stay up a bit late	Bright light in the morning
Sleep a bit late	Go to bed early
Bright light in the evening	Wake up early
Day of flight	During flight
Enjoy caffeine	Avoid caffeine
After arrival	After arrival
Get bright light in the evening	Get outdoors early in the morning
Dark sunglasses in the morning	

Although surprising, sleep deprivation is useful in depression, despite the fact that depressed patients most commonly complain of trouble sleeping and often request sedatives. There is no evidence that hypnotics add to the treatment of depression; indeed, an early report suggests that a triple combination of sleep deprivation, bright light treatment, and antidepressants may produce particularly dramatic improvement *(6)*.

4. LIGHT TREATMENT FOR JET LAG AND SHIFT WORK

Short jet flights across one to six time zones produce a "jet-lag" syndrome quite similar to advanced or delayed sleep-phase, where the body clock phase becomes inappropriate for the new time zone. The treatments are similar. Table 3 lists some of the principles. The treatments here might seem simple, compared to the multitudes of remedies purported to be treatments, such as special diets. Nonetheless, these suggestions are based on scientifically proven principles.

4.1. Flying East

Flights east of up to six time zones, for example, from Los Angeles to New York or from Chicago to London, produce a condition quite similar to a delayed sleep-phase. The traveler will experience trouble falling asleep at a convenient hour in the new time zone and trouble awakening early enough the next morning. For such flights, adjustment will be encouraged by using bright light for a day or two before the flight as early in the morning as possible, bright light on the morning of the flight, and bright light if possible for a morning or two after arrival. When adjusting to the anticipated flight in advance, it is useful to retire and get up early for a day or two in combination with using the bright morning light. Reducing caffeine use on the day of the flight will probably be helpful.

For east-going flights of more than six time zones, for example, for the flight from Los Angeles to Paris or from Hong Kong to San Francisco, the use of bright morning light could be counterproductive. Currently, we do not understand either the human phase-response curve or the practical experience of jet travelers well enough to be certain what will be helpful for very long east-going flights, especially those which go overnight.

4.2. West-Going Flights

Flying west, from New York to Los Angeles or from Los Angeles to Tokyo, for example, produces a circadian phase disturbance quite similar to an advanced sleep-phase. For such flights, getting bright light for an evening or two before the flight and an evening or two after is helpful. For a day or two after the flight, also, getting outdoors for a time just before sundown may be particularly useful, whereas heavy sunglasses should be worn when going outdoors in the morning. Caffeine may be particularly helpful during adjustment to west-going flights.

Using evening light will probably be helpful for west-going flights across up to ten time zones, but beyond ten time zones, the effects of light may be less predictable.

4.3. Bright Light for Night Shift Workers

As predicted from our knowledge of the circadian phase-response curve, initial studies suggest that bright light helps workers adjust to the switch to night-shift work. Unfortunately, these studies have generally involved only a few nights of night-shift work. Whether bright light will be useful for the worker who does night-shifts week after week remains to be demonstrated, because the benefits of adjusting to night work might be balanced by greater difficulty adjusting to days off. Therefore, the use of bright light for shift workers seems rather experimental, however promising.

5. TECHNICAL CONSIDERATIONS
IN APPLYING BRIGHT LIGHT THERAPY

Brightness is one of the most important factors in successful light treatment, in addition to timing and duration. So far as we know, both ceiling lighting and eye-level lighting work equally. As far as we know, sunlight and artificial lighting work equally well, and incandescent and fluorescent lighting work equally well. Some people are annoyed by the flicker and sound of fluorescents, but fluorescent fixtures with electronic (high frequency) ballasts will probably cause less headache and eye strain. There are two important advantages of fluorescent fixtures. First, since fluorescent lighting is more energy-efficient, it requires less electricity and produces less wasted heat. That heat could be annoying in the summer. Second, fluorescent tubes are large, so it is easy to diffuse the light over an area of several square feet. This means that unlike the very bright point of light produced by incandescent bulbs, fluorescents produce somewhat dimmer light over a larger area. When the light goes through the lens of the eye and hits the retina, the energy of the diffused light is spread over a larger area, so that it is less likely to burn the retina or to cause visual spots (like the spots seen after looking at a flash bulb). As a general rule, a patient cannot burn the retina by staring at any of the common fluorescent bulbs or diffusers, even receiving 10,000 lux, but it is less certain that staring at certain incandescent bulbs is entirely within the range of safety.

Indirect incandescent lighting should be safe. The problem with indirect incandescent lighting for treating depression is that the standard commercial lamps lose most of the brightness by bouncing the light off the walls and ceiling, partly because the light travels a greater distance. As a result, the lighting store incandescent lamps are probably not bright enough to do the job well for depression, although as discussed above, they might be sufficient for most cases of advanced sleep-phase. Another problem is that 300- to 500-watt halogen incandescent bulbs do not last very long and may be a bit difficult to replace. For these reasons, all of the lighting fixtures that I can currently recommend (at least for depression) use fluorescent bulbs and diffusers.

Several manufacturers make fluorescent fixtures that do a very nice job of helping depressed patients. (*See* Chapter 10, Appendix 2, for a list of bright light box manufacturers.) In general, 200- to 300-watts of fluorescent light illuminating a bright diffuser about one yard from the eyes will give about 2000 to 3000 lux. The exact brightness depends on various aspects such as the bulbs, the diffusers, and the reflectors. To get 10,000 lux, the manufacturers may recommend a somewhat bigger fixture with more wattage and also placing the fixture closer to the eyes, perhaps 12 to 18 inches. Some of the designs hold the light tilted a bit above the eyes, which seems to be convenient for giving light treatment and allowing writing, eating, or watching TV at the same time.

Some researchers have recommended that people stare at the fluorescent diffuser most of the time they are getting the treatment; others have recommended glancing at the light every minute or two. Others seem to feel that having the light source anywhere in the field of vision (even if not looking at it directly) is just as good. Unfortunately, we do not know yet whether it makes much difference whether the patient looks directly at the lighting. Most evidence suggests that having the light within the field of vision and glancing at it occasionally is sufficient. Unfortunately, we also really do not know if it makes a difference where the light is during treatment: above the eyes (tilted), straight out, to the side, or even below where the person is looking.

Much has been written about natural lighting and whether one should use lighting with a "full" spectrum. Most of the claims lack scientific basis. In fact, the FDA forced one company advertising "full spectrum" light into a consent decree admitting that their claims were deceptive. Almost any white light produces the full visible spectrum of colors (light wave lengths). The question is the balance of the different wavelengths, which does differ from one light source to another. If one looks at the fine spectrum with a precision spectrophotometer, few commercial sources really produce a light spectrum which could be mistaken for the rather smooth spectrum of natural sunlight. Fortunately, the eye is not a spectrophotometer, and there is no evidence that sunlight is necessary. The main issue is how much ultraviolet light the light source produces, because some of the "full spectrum" bulbs give off enough ultraviolet to possibly increase cataracts or skin cancer. There is no evidence that the ultraviolet is needed for the bright light treatment benefit; consequently I do not recommend anything with significant ultraviolet content. Most of the fluorescent manufacturers use a plastic diffuser which filters out the harmful ultraviolet. Appendix 2 in Chapter 10 lists some of the manufacturers.

5.2. Case Study

A 60-year-old man presented with the complaint of difficulty getting to sleep each evening because of restless legs. His schedule was that at about 10 PM (PST) each evening, he began to get a restless feeling in the thighs if he lay down and tried to sleep. This had been present for many years, and he coped with it by sitting up in the evenings, working at his desk or computer, and doing little chores. Over time, he developed a pattern of staying up very late at night to avoid going to sleep, and also drinking two to three ounces of brandy to help induce sleep by about 2 or 3 AM. Because he slept best in the morning hours, and because he was self-employed as a writer and consultant, he was able to sleep late each morning. However, recent changes in his business necessitated meetings or phone calls with the east coast, preferably before 9 AM PST. When he was getting up, usually at about 11 AM or noon, he would tend to avoid going outside, and begin to work again in his home.

He denied any general medical diseases and had a full physical evaluation for life insurance about two years earlier. He admitted to general mild discouragement over his insomnia and fatigue but denied feeling depressed or irritable. He did not have changes in appetite or weight.

There was no significant past medical history. He smoked about a pack of cigarets per day. He took no medications.

The physical examination was remarkable for a somewhat gaunt and pale man, who seemed fatigued. The examination was conducted at 10 AM, about the time he would be waking up. Vital signs were normal, and the general physical examination was normal. The neurological examination suggested mild decreased sensation in the feet, but was otherwise negative. The mental status was normal, but he presented mild generalized slowness of speech and response to questions. Range of affect was somewhat diminished. He was fully oriented with no evidence of psychosis.

The diagnoses of restless legs syndrome and delayed sleep-phase syndrome were made, and the patient was started on Sinemet (25/100) each evening. He was told to discontinue alcohol after dinner. He was given information on circadian rhythms, and told to get up at 10 AM each morning and go outside for a walk of at least 30 minutes duration. Two weeks later, he reported that the Sinemet at about 11 PM had helped his legs, and he was more comfortable each evening and nighttime. He had stopped alcohol without problem and felt somewhat more productive in the evenings. However, he had not gotten up at any particular time, and he did not feel capable of going for a walk each day. He remained unable to fall asleep before 2 or 3 AM. The importance of the morning wake-up time and morning bright light was re-emphasized, and he agreed to set an alarm for 10:30, be outside within to sit on his porch within 30 minutes, for at least 30 minutes. He would then reset the time of the alarm and porch sitting 30 minutes earlier every 3 days up to 9 AM, and we agreed that a sleeping time of 1 AM to 9 AM would be the goal. Two weeks later, he was able to accomplish the wake-up times with the use of the alarm but felt worse overall—he did not like going outside and still had trouble falling asleep before 2 or 3 AM. A bright light box was prescribed and the patient purchased a commercial model. He continued the wake-up time of 9 AM and then used a bright light box at the breakfast table and on his work desk from about 9:30 AM until 11:30 AM. Within a few days, he found it easier to fall asleep, and with the Sinemet taken at about 11 PM, could fall asleep at 1 AM. He felt more alert and productive in the morning hours than before, and was pleased with his new ability to control both the restless legs and his sleep onset times. He has continued to use this regimen for 3 years.

REFERENCES

1. Arendt J. *Melatonin and the Mammalian Pineal Gland*. London, Chapman & Hall, 1995, pp. 1–331.
2. Campbell SS, Dawson D, Anderson MW. Alleviation of sleep maintenance insomnia with timed exposure to bright light. *J Am Geriatr Soc* 1993; 41: 829–836.
3. Kripke DF, Youngstedt SD. Illumination levels in wake and sleep, in *Biologic Effects of Light 1995* (Holick, MF, Jung EG, eds), Walter de Gruyter, Berlin, 1996, pp. 332–339.
4. Avery DH, Bolte MA, Dager SR, Wilson LG, Weyer M, Cox GB, Dunner DL. Dawn simulation treatment of winter depression: A controlled study. *Am J Psych* 1993; 150: 113–117.
5. Schwartz PJ, Brown C, Wehr TA, Rosenthal NE. Winter seasonal affective disorder: A follow-up study of the first 59 patients of the National Institute of Mental Health Seasonal Studies Program. *Am J Psych* 1996; 153: 1028–1036.
6. Neumeister A, Goessler R, Lucht M, Kapitany T, Bamas C, Kasper S. Bright light therapy stabilizes the antidepressant effect of partial sleep deprivation. *Biol Psych* 1996; 39: 16–21.

4

Restless Legs Syndrome
and Nocturnal Myoclonus

J. Steven Poceta

Contents

1. INTRODUCTION

Restless legs syndrome (RLS) was first described by Dr. Karl Ekbom in 1945 in his article "Restless legs." The condition is usually associated with periodic limb movements in sleep (PLMS). PLMS is also called nocturnal myoclonus. The vast majority of patients with RLS also have PLMS, but many patients exhibit PLMS without having RLS. Restless legs syndrome is not an uncommon cause of insomnia, and is receiving more and more public attention. A national RLS Foundation has been formed, which is assisting local patient support groups around the country and is raising funds for research.

2. CLINICAL PRESENTATIONS

The complaints offered by patients with RLS will fall into one or more of the following broad categories: 1) unpleasant physical sensa-

From: *Sleep Disorders: Diagnosis and Treatment*
Edited by: J. S. Poceta and M. M. Mitler © Humana Press Inc., Totowa, NJ

Restless legs syndrome and PLMS are:

- often coexistent.
- distinguished by the fact that RLS is diagnosed based on subjective sensations, and PLMS is diagnosed on the basis of observed movements during sleep.
- common causes of sleep complaints, especially in the elderly.

tions, 2) insomnia, 3) daytime sleepiness, and 4) nocturnal movements. Of course, physical sensations, insomnia, and sleepiness are all subjective symptoms which are difficult to quantitate, and which often do not correlate well with objective measures. Restless legs syndrome should be considered in any patient with one of these symptoms.

Unpleasant physical sensations refers to the major symptom of RLS, which is a hard-to-describe feeling that makes the patient want to move the legs. Often, there is a somatic sensation such as tingling or deep itching in addition to the more general feelings of restlessness. Sometimes, the patient might deny a feeling of restlessness itself, except insofar as the unpleasant feeling is briefly relieved by moving. Words such as creepy-crawly, worms under the skin, itching, or electricity are sometimes used to describe the sensation. Most patients will deny that the feeling is painful, even though it is extremely unpleasant. I often ask patients what would happen if they tried to force themselves not to move the legs. Many patients say that they would "go crazy," and give in to the feeling to move. Some say that in addition, the feeling would build up and result in an involuntary jerk or twitch.

The sensation is usually located in the lower extremities, but the exact location varies from patient to patient. In most cases, the sensation is not primarily located in the toes or feet, as might be expected in neuropathy. The calves and thighs, either anterior or posterior, or throughout, are most common. RLS should be bilateral but occasionally will be worse on one side. In rare cases, the primary location is the arms, the trunk, or generalized throughout the body. At least two factors contribute to the intensity of the RLS sensation: the activity of the patient and the time of day. Most patients will not be bothered by RLS when they are active or moving about, but the feeling occurs when they are sedentary, usually sitting or reclining. Independent of the activity of the patient is the circadian timing of the severity of RLS, with evenings and nights being worse than early morning and daytime.

Patients with restless legs syndrome or PLMS usually present one or more of the following complaints:

- unpleasant physical sensations in the legs.
- insomnia, usually sleep onset or sleep maintenance.
- daytime sleepiness and nonrestorative sleep.
- restless sleep and nocturnal movements, often noticed mostly by the bedpartner.

The circadian timing of the RLS sensation and the usual relaxing and sedentary activities near bedtime often cause an inability to initiate or maintain sleep, thus resulting in the symptom of insomnia. Sometimes, patients are not aware of a specific sensation in the legs, but simply "toss and turn" for long periods of time when trying to initiate or return to sleep. These patients may think that their insomnia is nonspecific, caused by stress, or an inability to "turn off the mind." Thus, RLS and PLMS need to be considered in any patient complaining of insomnia. Once asleep, some patients are aware that a jerk of the legs in sleep awakened them, and then restlessness will not allow them to return to sleep. Interestingly, many patients with RLS obtain their best sleep in the early morning hours (e.g., 5 AM), and some develop a tendency to a delayed sleep phase.

Daytime sleepiness can result from the sleep disruption caused by RLS and PLMS. However, it is unusual for patients with RLS to have no complaint of insomnia but to have daytime sleepiness. On the other hand, PLMS alone can produce repetitive brief arousals during sleep of which the patient is unaware, and thus produce daytime sleepiness or nonrestorative sleep. Patients with RLS can thus present with sleepiness or nonrestorative sleep on the basis of insufficient total sleep time or poor quality sleep.

A fourth type of presenting complaint might come from the bedpartner. It is not unusual for the bedpartner to notice the repetitive and periodic movements during sleep in patients with PLMS. Sometimes, these movements are vigorous enough to keep the bedpartner awake or cause him or her to sleep in a different room for years before seeking medical help. Sometimes, the patients will not have any specific complaints about restlessness, insomnia, or sleepiness but will give the history that they sleep best in unusual settings, such as on the floor, in part because of excessive movements in the bed that disturb the bedpartner.

Table 1
Diagnostic Criteria for Restless Legs Syndrome

1. Desire to move the extremities, often associated with paresthesias or dysesthesia. These dysesthesia can be variably described as "creeping" or "tingling."
2. Motor restlessness.
3. The symptoms are partially and briefly relieved by movement, and worsened at rest.
4. The symptoms worsen in the evening or night.
5. Polysomnographic monitoring usually demonstrates PLMS.

Table 2
Description of PLMS

1. A complaint of insomnia or excessive sleepiness, or movements noticed by an observer.
2. Repetitive limb muscle movements, which in the leg are characterized by dorsiflexion of the great toe and ankle, in combination with partial flexion of the knee, and sometimes the hip.
3. Polysomnography demonstrates: Repetitive episodes of muscle contraction (0.5–5 seconds in duration) separated by an interval of typically 20–40 seconds, and arousals or awakenings may be associated with the movements.

Accepted diagnostic criteria for RLS are given in Table 1. In essence, the patient should describe an unpleasant but not painful feeling of restlessness or creeping within the extremities. This feeling should be briefly relieved with movement, and the patient should exhibit motor restlessness. This restlessness can take the form of tossing and turning when awake or dozing in bed, pacing, exercising, shaking of the limbs, or rubbing the limbs. The symptoms should worsen at rest and be partially relieved with movement. They should also predominate in the evening and night hours.

Table 2 describes PLMS. Figure 1 shows their periodic nature as measured on a polysomnogram. However, it must be noted that there is controversy as to the significance of PLMS when it is not associated with restless legs, insomnia, poor quality sleep, or daytime sleepiness. Epidemiologic studies have shown that these repetitive movements are present in as many as 44% of senior citizens in the United States. Thus, complaints of PLMS noticed by a bedpartner but in the absence of complaints from the patient might be less significant and might not need to be treated.

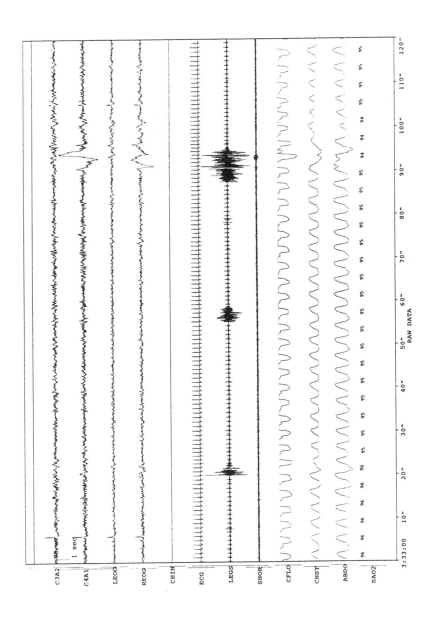

Fig. 1. Nocturnal myoclonus on overnight polysomnogram. Note the obvious potentials coming from the leg EMG channel, which are caused by anterior tibialis contraction and associated with movement of the ankles and legs. There is associated EEG arousal with the third contraction in this example.

79

RLS is a syndrome, not a specific disease, because:

- RLS is an aggregate of symptoms.
- There is no known, identifiable etiologic agent.
- Identification of a specific cause is possible only in a minority of cases.

3. ETIOLOGY AND PATHOPHYSIOLOGY

There is no established etiology of restless legs syndrome or of PLMS. A majority of cases are idiopathic. However, we can extrapolate as to potential causative factors given the association of RLS with certain other diseases and the effectiveness of certain medications.

3.1. Genetics

A positive family history is reported in as many as one-third to one-half of patients with RLS. In the few large kindreds studied, an autosomal dominant mode of inheritance has been suggested. However, no linkage studies have yet identified a specific gene or chromosome. There is a suggestion that younger and more severely affected patients more often report affected family members. However, since some surveys have indicated that as many as 10% of the population might have symptoms compatible with RLS, genetic surveys will need to take into account the common nature of this condition.

3.2. Neurochemical Hypotheses

There are data to suggest that central nervous system dopamine plays a role in RLS. First, dopaminergic medications are often highly effective in treating the sensations of RLS. Sinemet (carbidopa/levodopa), a dopamine precursor which increases synaptic dopamine, is well documented to decrease both the symptoms of RLS and to suppress PLMS. Dopamine agonists such as pergolide and bromocriptine are also effective. Secondly, there appears to be an increase in the occurrence of PLMS in patients with Parkinson's Disease, and restlessness is often a symptom when dopamine effect is waning. However, we are not aware that there is an increased incidence of Parkinson's Disease in patients who present with RLS. Finally, one study utilized single photon emission tomography in 20 patients with PLMS and demonstrated decreased dopamine receptor occupancy in the central nervous system.

Opiates such as codeine, propoxyphene, and methadone are also effective in treating RLS, suggesting an alteration of central endorphin systems. Their effect is probably not related solely to the analgesic effect of the drugs, since these agents also decrease the number of leg movements in patients with PLMS.

3.3. Alterations in the Sensory Nervous System

Because of the nature of the sensation and the movements in RLS, it seems obvious that some abnormality of the nervous system underlies this condition, particularly the sensory nervous system. Because the sensation is primarily in the legs, RLS has some clinical similarities to peripheral neuropathy. Indeed, one study of 154 patients with polyneuropathy found that 5.2% had symptoms of RLS. Thus, there is a relationship between peripheral neuronal degeneration and RLS, but it is not a universal relationship in all patients. Some have also noticed a relation between lumbar spinal disease and RLS. Others have found that removal of painful varicose veins in the legs can ameliorate RLS. Some have advocated that cold feet associated with arterial insufficiency is associated with RLS. Many of these conditions that seem to have a relation to RLS have in common an alteration of the peripheral nervous system— either at the level of the spinal nerves or more distal. Thus, one can postulate that RLS arises in a susceptible individual in whom an insult of some kind occurs to alter sensory input from the legs into the central nervous system. There, modulation of this input somehow produces the unusual phenomenon of restlessness. Obviously, more data is needed to explain fully the syndrome, especially its marked circadian tendencies.

4. ASSOCIATED CONDITIONS AND FINDINGS

4.1. Iron Deficiency Anemia and Gastric Surgeries

There are several lines of evidence that show that iron deficiency anemia sometimes causes RLS and PLMS. In one early series by Ekbom, RLS was common in a series of patients who had undergone gastric surgeries and who presumably had one or more vitamin or mineral deficiencies, including iron deficiency. More recent series have demonstrated that in a series of randomly selected geriatric patients admitted to a hospital in the UK, the complaint of restless legs was significantly correlated with certain measures of iron deficiency, most notably a low ferritin. In other patient populations, iron is increasingly associated with neurocognitive conditions. For example, it has been observed that neuroleptic-induced akithesia can be modified by concomitant administration of iron is some hospitalized psychiatric patients.

The pathophysiologic mechanism by which iron deficiency could produce a symptom such as restlessness, and why it does so only in certain individuals, is not known. Iron is one of the more abundant minerals in the brain and is involved in mitochondrial function in dopamine-producing neurons. Iron is also a component of the central dopamine receptors in the basal ganglia. Besides a direct effect of iron on neuronal function and central dopamine systems, the possibility also exists that the decreased oxygen carrying capacity of the blood is somehow involved in producing RLS in these patients.

4.2. Uremia

The occurrence of PLMS is well known in patients with renal failure, especially those on hemodialysis. There are also reports of improvement in RLS and PLMS with administration of levodopa in patients on hemodialysis. The mechanism is unknown, and it is also not known if there is an association with the anemia of renal failure. PLMS should be considered as a specific cause of insomnia in such patients.

4.3. Neuropathy

Many of the features of RLS are also present in peripheral neuropathy. Although there are many differences, it is not always easy to distinguish dysesthesias as being from a peripheral neuropathy as opposed to RLS. The sensations are usually in the legs; sometimes described as numbness or tingling and are often worse at night and at rest. Thus, peripheral neuropathy must be considered in the differential diagnosis of leg pains or leg complaints. As mentioned above, the conditions coexist, and thus it seems that peripheral neuropathy can be a cause of RLS. In fact, Ekbom noted that up to 17% of patients with diabetes (who presumably had a degree of peripheral neuropathy) complained of restless legs. In addition to the association of RLS with peripheral neuropathy, there is also evidence that RLS itself is a manifestation of a subclinical neuropathy. One study in 1995 found evidence of axonal neuropathy in eight of eight patients, when studied with either nerve biopsy or nerve conduction/electromyogram. None of these patients had bedside evidence of neuropathy, and the significance of this finding is not yet clear, except that peripheral neuropathy should be considered in any patient presenting with RLS.

4.4. Spinal Cord Disease and Miscellaneous Conditions

There are scattered reports of lumbar radiculopathy, low back pain, and myelopathy causing or contributing to RLS. The true contribution of these conditions to RLS and PLMS is not clear, but clinical experience suggests that a significant proportion of RLS patients have spinal cord disease. RLS and PLMS have also been reported as possibly more common in amyloidosis, chronic lung diseases, leukemias, rheumatoid arthritis, and fibromyalgia. In addition, certain medications can precipitate RLS or induce PLMS. Most notably are certain antidepressants, both the tricyclics and the serotonin re-uptake inhibitors, such as fluoxetine and paroxetine.

4.5. Other Sleep Disorders

PLMS has been reported to be more common in patients with obstructive sleep apnea (OSA) or narcolepsy. There might be an underlying pathophysiology by which these conditions, by impacting the sleep–wake mechanisms of the brain, could produce PLMS. It is also commonly observed that RLS and PLMS worsen in association with poor sleep from any cause. For example, when sleep is disrupted by anxiety or mental stress, RLS symptoms are worse. We have seen cases of severe RLS and PLMS exacerbated by symptoms of congestive heart failure, including Cheyne-Stokes periodic breathing. Treatment of the CHF greatly improved the RLS sensations and overall sleep quality.

Thus, RLS and PLMS often coexist with other sleep disorders, including narcolepsy, sleep-disordered breathing, and REM behavior disorder. REM behavior disorder is a recently described condition in which patients are physically active during their dreams. The condition is not rare, is most common in older men, and is particularly common in certain neurodegenerative conditions such as Parkinson's Disease and multisystem atrophy. Most cases are idiopathic. A majority of patients with REM behavior disorder have significant PLMS. The bedpartner will report activity during periods of sleep in which the patient appears to be dreaming. Typically, there will be talking, twitching, jerking, or more semipurposeful movements such as punching, kicking, or picking. If awakened, the patient will usually report a vivid dream, sometimes violent and usually active, and consistent with the observed behavior. A neurologic evaluation is desirable in such cases to rule out a concomitant condition. Klonopin (clonazepam) in low doses at bedtimes is remarkably effective for REM behavior disorder.

5. DIFFERENTIAL DIAGNOSTIC CONSIDERATIONS

There are three aspects to the consideration of the correct diagnosis of RLS and PLMS. The first is to determine that the patient has RLS and/or PLMS and not some other condition mimicking it. For example, several conditions produce unpleasant leg or limb sensations. Peripheral neuropathy tends to produce a tingling or burning numbness beginning distally in the foot, which can be worse in the night. Lumbar

Table 3
Differential Diagnosis and Associated Conditions

RLS and PLMS must be differentiated from
  1. Hypnic jerks.
  2. Myoclonic epilepsy.
  3. Peripheral neuropathy and lumbar radiculopathy.
  4. Sleep-disordered breathing.
RLS and PLMS can be caused by
  1. Iron-deficiency anemia.
  2. Uremia.
  3. Peripheral neuropathy.
  4. Lumbar or spinal cord disease.

radiculopathy can produce leg aching. Spasticity can also produce unpleasant leg sensations and even "jerks"; consequently myelopathy must be sought for carefully. Myoclonic epilepsy can also produce jerks that have a circadian pattern. Repetitive jerks at sleep onset are quite common and are normal. Erythromelalgia (aching painful distal legs from edema) has some characteristics that are similar to RLS. Lastly, leg aching from poor physical conditioning, sedentary lifestyle, and even excessive caffeine use can mimic RLS. PLMS can cause repeated jerking in sleep with arousal, a nonspecific complaint that can be found in other sleep disorders, most notably sleep apnea. In some patients with sleep apnea, even severe OSA, the patient and bedpartner are aware primarily of the arousal phase of the process, at which time there might be rather prominent movement and jerking of the limbs (Table 3). Secondly, after one is fairly confident that the complaint is consistent with RLS or PLMS, potential causative conditions should be considered. Conditions such as iron deficiency anemia, peripheral neuropathy, lumbar spine disease, and uremia have been enumerated above.

Finally, even when one is confident that RLS and/or PLMS are present in a patient, and even after associated conditions have been sought for and perhaps identified, there remains the issue of whether RLS/PLMS is responsible for the person's complaint. This is a particularly difficult issue in patients who do not have RLS but have a chief complaint of insomnia or nonrestorative sleep, and who are determined by observation or by sleep study (polysomnogram) to have PLMS. The complaint of insomnia is commonly caused by stress, anxiety, depression, poor sleep hygiene and some lifestyles. PLMS is often an incidental finding in normal sleepers, especially the elderly. Thus, the relationship of PLMS to complaint is not always certain, and can be one of degree. Clinical judgment and medication trials must be utilized.

When evaluating symptoms which could indicate RLS or PLMS, consider:

- Are these symptoms consistent only with RLS/PLMS, or with other conditions?
- If RLS/PLMS can be diagnosed, can a cause of the syndrome be identified?
- If RLS/PLMS can be diagnosed, how much does it contribute to the patient's complaints and problems (how significant is it)?

6. MEDICAL EVALUATION AND WORK-UP

6.1. Findings on Physical Examination

By definition, the physical examination is normal in patients with RLS. However, the physical examination may be abnormal in cases in which the RLS is associated with another condition, such as peripheral neuropathy. A detailed neurologic examination should be performed in patients suspected of having RLS or PLMS in order both to verify the diagnosis and to identify potentially causative conditions. Signs of myelopathy, radiculopathy, peripheral neuropathy, congestive heart failure, and arthritis in particular should be investigated.

Any patient with RLS and/or PLMS should be screened with blood tests to include electrolytes, blood urea nitrogen and creatinine, complete blood count with red cell indices, serum ferritin, and thyroid function tests. Additional studies to include potential causes of neuropathy, such as serum protein electrophoresis and B-12 level are reasonable.

The decision to refer a patient with suspected RLS or PLMS to a sleep specialist must be made by the primary care physician based on his or her experience, resources, and the desires of the patient. Obviously, the level of comfort of the primary physician as to certainty of diagnosis and treatment regimens is the main consideration. The specialist is likely to be in the best position to confirm the specific diagnosis and whether any sleep studies or neurophysiologic studies such as EEG are indicated prior to initiation of treatment. The suspicion of a coexisting disease such as OSA would be one important reason to perform to overnight polysomnography or at least some screening for OSA. In general, milder cases which are well treated with intermittent use of a benzodiazepine (e.g., clonazepam or temazepam) probably do not need referral. However, when the primary care physician is faced with a patient who has significant complaints (e.g., daytime sleepiness, or a patient who is not responding well to treatment, or a patient who is using escalating doses of medications, referral is indicated.

7. TREATMENT CONSIDERATIONS

Although many treatments have been tried for RLS, over time, three categories of drugs have been consistently helpful: benzodiazepines, opiates, and dopaminergic agents.

7.1. Benzodiazepines

Several of these sedative–hypnotic agents have been shown in both double-blind studies and clinical experience to improve sleep by decreasing arousals and to some extent decreasing leg jerks. Studies indicate that, in general, the benzodiazepines are more useful as sedatives than as treatments for the RLS sensation itself or for the limb movements. Thus, they are probably most likely to be useful in those patients with insomnia as the chief component of their syndrome. Clonazepam (Klonopin) is perhaps the best known agent, but diazepam (Valium), temazepam (Restoril), and triazolam (Halcion) have all been shown to be effective. The choice of the agent often depends more on the pharmacokinetic and side effect profiles than on any specific aspect of the drug. However, clinical experience does seem to suggest that there is something different about clonazepam, such that its effect on muscle and limb jerking is more pronounced. The benzodiazepines can all produce dependency, and tolerance with dose-escalation can be a problem. In addition, these agents are sometimes poorly tolerated, especially when in the elderly, they produce excessive or prolonged sedation. Nocturnal confusion and ataxia have been encountered. Nonetheless, in younger patients with insomnia as a result of PLMS or RLS, the benzodiazepines might be considered first line therapy.

7.2. Opiates

Ekbom used codeine to treat some of his patients; even today, the opioid mediations remain useful. A limited number of studies have shown that certain of these agents have a mild to moderate effect on the number of leg jerks, the severity of the restlessness, and the quality of the sleep. In general, they are not as effective as the benzodiazepines for sedation or the dopaminergics for control of the restlessness. Nonetheless, many patients benefit from their use. Codeine, propoxyphene, and oxycodone are the most commonly prescribed. In some patients, methadone is necessary. Side effects include constipation, confusion, and the problems of dependency and tolerance. Without question, there are some patients who are able to use low or moderate doses for years without tolerance or dose escalation. Unfortunately, there are also patients who develop these problems, even to the point of dependency and drug-seeking behaviors. Since RLS symptoms, insomnia, pain, and anxiety often interact in patients, careful monitoring of these medications is necessary.

7.3. Dopaminergics

L-Dopa is a precursor to dopamine, which enhances neuronal dopamine synthesis and release. In the 1980s L-Dopa with a decarboxylase inhibitor (Sinemet in the US) was noted to relieve many of the symptoms of RLS. Since then, several studies have proven its effect for both short-term and long-term treatment of the condition. As many as 70% of patients with RLS obtain relief by taking Sinemet. The effect is rapid, usually within 30–60 minutes after ingestion. Sinemet and its generics have an effect lasting two to four hours, but the controlled release (CR) form of the medication can produce effect up to six hours, accomplished by slowing gastrointestinal breakdown of the pill itself, thus prolonging intestinal absorption. Sinemet is not only effective in relieving the RLS, but also decreases the PLMS. Thus, sleep onset and sleep maintenance can be improved by the use of this agent. Research studies have shown, however, that Sinemet does not decrease arousals associated with the leg jerks, a finding that contradicts much clinical experience. Sinemet can be considered the agent of first choice when the target symptoms are those of RLS, and especially when patient considerations make the problems of benzodiazepines and opiates undesirable. For instance, Sinemet is an ideal first choice in patients with RLS who are over the age of 60 years or have had previous complications of sedative or narcotic use. Clearly, the use of Sinemet or any dopaminergic agent must be considered "off-label." Whereas the use of certain benzodiazepines is approved and indicated by the FDA for insomnia, and the use of narcotics is approved and indicated for pain conditions (which patients with RLS can be considered as having), none of the dopaminergic agents have any similar labeling. Thus, some primary care physicians prefer to leave prescription of the dopaminergic agents to the specialist.

Side effects of L-Dopa include nausea, dizziness, or nightmares and, occasionally, confusion. The drug is remarkably well tolerated in this (nonParkinson) population and in doses usually under 600 mg per day. The side effects common to the Parkinson patient taking higher doses such as abnormal involuntary movements or hallucinations have not been observed. However, as many as 50% of RLS patients who initially benefit from Sinemet will develop certain problems. The most common

In addition to medications aimed at minimizing RLS and PLMS, it is also important to:

- Emphasize good sleep hygiene such as a regular morning wakeup time, exercise, and sunlight exposure.
- Educate the patient in appropriate goals, and the fact that these conditions are often chronic and incurable, although the symptoms can be minimized.
- Consider, evaluate and treat other conditions which can cause sleep disturbance, especially anxiety, depression, conditioned insomnia, and sleep apnea.

is that of a shifting in the timing of the RLS symptoms. For example, a patient who was suffering from RLS from 10 PM until midnight might normally begin taking Sinemet at 9 or 10 PM. After a period of a few weeks, the patient might begin to notice that the RLS is now occurring at 7 or 8 PM. Sometimes medication at that earlier time is needed, and as a result a few patients need to take Sinemet around the clock. This is usually not desirable because it is not often effective—patients get symptoms before the next dose; also, the generally higher total daily doses increase the risk of toxicity. Other complications include a worsening of the intensity of the RLS sensation in the before-dose period, and/or movement of the sensation to other body parts, such as the trunk or arms. Usually, Sinemet will need to be discontinued in patients with such problems, and other dopaminergic agents might then be tried.

Parlodel (bromocriptine) and Permax (pergolide) are direct dopamine receptor agonists both of which can be quite helpful to the patient with RLS. They tend to have slower dose onset than L-Dopa, and have longer biologic activity. They do not involve stimulation of dopamine production. These agents do not seem to produce the rebound effects of L-Dopa. Either can be administered near bedtime only, or twice, such as at dinner and at bedtime. The timing of the doses are determined by the timing of target symptoms. Although less well studied than L-Dopa, they are clearly effective in a majority of RLS patients. Permax seems to be the most widely used. Newer dopamine agonists (pramipexole and ropinerol) are not yet tested in patients with RLS, but early clinical experience suggests efficacy, especially with pramipexole.

A variety of other treatments are sometimes used. As one might expect from a subjective problem such as RLS, especially one in which there can be considerable variation from night-to-night and year-to-year, many patients will develop idiosyncratic treatment concepts. Vitamin E

tive heart failure. There was no evidence of weakness. There was mild depression of each ankle jerk (Achilles tendon jerk). About two years previously, blood chemistries, CBC, TSH, B-12 level, and serum iron were all normal.

She was treated with carbidopa/levodopa, 25/100 mg tablets, taken in the late evening about one hour before bedtime. She experienced significant lessening of the restless sensation beginning about 45 minutes after she took the pill. She was able to fall asleep much more quickly and slept more continuously for the first couple hours of the night. She experienced no side effects. She was changed to the 25/100 Sinemet CR taken at about the same time to prolong the effect and began to sleep better throughout the night. Evening restlessness was treated intermittently, as needed, with one-half or one tablet of the regular 25/100.

Follow-up 14 months later revealed that she continued to benefit. She was aware of some mild increase in the intensity of her restlessness in the early evening, but it was easily managed by distraction, and she continued to sleep well. Her total daily dose of levodopa remained at 200 mg. Ophthalmologic examination revealed no increase in intraocular pressure, and liver function studies were normal. She continues on levodopa.

Discussion

This lady illustrates some of the common features of RLS that are described above in the chapter. Her RLS was associated with lumbar radiculopathy and seemed to be triggered by it. She did well on levodopa both initially and apparently for the long-term, with no ill effects. When on levodopa chronically, intraocular pressure and liver function studies should probably be checked occasionally.

REFERENCES

1. Silber MH. Concise review for primary-care physicians. *Mayo Clin Proc* 1997; 72: 261–264.
2. Walters AS, et al. Toward a better definition of the restless legs syndrome. *Movement Disorders* 1995; 10: 634–642.
3. Walters AS, Hening W, Rubinstein M, Chokroverty S. A clinical and polysomnographic comparison of neuroleptic-induced akathisia and the idiopathic restless legs syndrome. *Sleep* 1991; 14: 339–345.
4. O'Keeffe ST, Noel J, Lavan JN. Restless legs syndrome in the elderly. *Postgrad Med J* 1993; 69: 701–703.

5

Narcolepsy and Excessive Daytime Sleepiness

Rafael Pelayo and Christian Guilleminault

CONTENTS

1. INTRODUCTION

A patient with unexplained sleepiness or fatigue presenting in a primary care setting often poses both a diagnostic and therapeutic dilemma. The etiology of the sleepiness may not be readily apparent. The patient and the general public may be at risk of serious personal injury unless prompt treatment is initiated. The risk of injury creates for the practitioner significant medical and legal responsibilities. Of all the different causes of excessive daytime sleepiness, narcolepsy should always be considered. Historically, the word "narcolepsy" was first coined by Gélineau in 1880 to designate a pathological condition characterized by irresistible episodes of sleep of short duration recurring at close intervals. In the same paper, he wrote that attacks were sometimes accompanied by falls or "astasias." In the 1930s, Daniels emphasized the association of cataplexy, hypnagogic hallucinations, sleep paralysis,

From: *Sleep Disorders: Diagnosis and Treatment*
Edited by: J. S. Poceta and M. M. Mitler © Humana Press Inc., Totowa, NJ

and excessive daytime sleepiness. Calling these symptoms the "tetrad" of narcolepsy Yoss, Daly, and Vogel described sleep-onset rapid eye movement sleep (REM) in narcoleptic patients. In 1963, Rechtschaffen et al. reported sleep-onset REM periods in narcolepsy. Narcolepsy is a neurological syndrome that is characterized by abnormal sleep, including excessive daytime sleepiness often with disturbed nocturnal sleep and pathological manifestations of REM. The REM abnormalities include early REM during sleep onset and cataplexy. Cataplexy is an abrupt and reversible decrease or loss of muscle tone, most frequently elicited by emotion.

It is important to consider narcolepsy as a cause of daytime sleepiness, especially in young patients, because it can take up to 20 years between the initial onset of sleepiness and development of the full clinical syndrome. During this lapse of time, the patient may be mislabeled with a wide variety of diagnoses. The patient may be considered lazy, to have "chronic fatigue," or to be depressed. Prior to being correctly diagnosed, the patient may turn to illegal drugs such as "crank" amphetamine to combat the sleepiness.

Narcolepsy is not a rare condition. The prevalence of narcolepsy has been calculated at about 0.04% of the general population. Its prevalence was calculated as 0.05% in the San Francisco Bay area and 0.067% in the Los Angeles area. A wide range of narcolepsy prevalence has been reported depending on the ethnic group studied. The condition was thought to be much more common among the Japanese population than among the Israeli; however, the way these studies were done render them inconclusive. The definition of the syndrome was different in Japan, and the sample was inappropriate for extrapolation to the total population in Israel. Males are affected somewhat more often than are females; age at onset varies from childhood to the fifth decade, peaking in the second decade. Special circumstances, such as an abrupt change of sleep-wake schedule, head trauma, or a severe psychological stress (e.g., death of a relative or divorce), precede the occurrence of the first symptom in as many as one-half of all cases.

This chapter will review narcolepsy and other causes of excessive daytime sleepiness that might be encountered in a primary care setting.

2. CLINICAL PRESENTATION: SYMPTOMS, SIGNS, AND DIAGNOSIS

2.1. Narcolepsy

Narcolepsy can be thought of as a chronic neurological disorder in which the boundaries between the waking, sleeping, and dreaming brain

Table 1
Key Signs and Symptoms of Narcolepsy

Sleep attacks
Cataplexy
Hypnagogic hallucinations
Sleep paralysis
Nocturnal sleep disruption

are blurred. The awake narcoleptic will feel sleepy. The sleeping narcoleptic will have disturbed sleep caused by arousals. REM-like activity
such as cataplexy and dream imagery will interrupt the awake state.
Narcolepsy is characterized by a set of clinical symptoms that include
abnormal sleep features, overwhelming episodes of sleep, excessive
daytime somnolence (EDS), hypnagogic hallucinations, disturbed nocturnal sleep, sleep paralysis, and manifestations of paroxysmal muscu-
lar weakness (cataplexy) Table 1 provides the key signs and symptoms
of narcolepsy.

Unwanted episodes of sleep recur several times a day, not only under
favorable circumstances such as monotonous sedentary activity or after
a meal, but also in situations in which the subject is involved in a task.
The duration of the episode may vary from a few minutes, if the subject
is in an uncomfortable position, to over an hour, if the subject is reclining. Narcoleptics characteristically wake up from naps or sleep attacks
refreshed, and there is a variable length refractory period before the next
episode occurs.

Apart from sleep episodes, patients may feel abnormally drowsy.
They may be spending the day at an unpleasant level of low alertness
that is responsible for poor performance at work, memory lapses, and
even gestural or speech automatisms. This low alertness may persist,
despite the use of stimulant medication.

Cataplexy is an abrupt and reversible decrease or loss of muscle tone
associated with narcolepsy most frequently elicited by emotions such as
laughter or anger, surprise, or abrupt strain. It may involve certain
muscles (especially proximal) or the entire voluntary musculature. Most
typically, the jaw sags, the head falls forward, the arms drop to the side,
and the knees buckle. The severity and extent of cataplectic attacks can
vary from a state of absolute powerlessness, which seems to involve the
entire voluntary musculature, to a limited involvement of certain muscle
groups or to no more than a fleeting sensation of weakness extending
more or less throughout the body. Although the extraocular muscles are
supposedly not involved, weakness can occur, and the patient may com-

plain of blurred or double vision. Complete paralysis of extraocular muscles has never been reported, however, although the palpebral muscles may be affected. Speech may be impaired, and respiration may become irregular during an attack, which may be related to weakness of the abdominal muscles. Long diaphragmatic pauses have never been recorded, but short diaphragmatic pauses similar to those seen during nocturnal REM sleep can be noted. Complete loss of muscle tone, which results in a total collapse with risk of serious injuries, including skull and other bone fractures, may occur during a cataplectic attack. However, the attacks are usually not so dramatic, and can be so subtle that they go unnoticed by nearby individuals. An attack may consist only of a slight buckling of the knees. Patients may perceive this abrupt and short-lasting weakness and may simply stop or stand against a wall. The condition may be slightly more obvious when there is a combination of sagging jaw and inclined head. Speech may be broken, owing to intermittent weakness affecting the arytenoid muscles. As seen during nocturnal REM sleep, the abrupt muscle inhibition is interrupted by sudden bursts of returning muscle tone, which, at times, even seems enhanced. If the weakness involves only the jaw or speech, the subject may present with wide masticatory movement or a weird attack of stuttering. If it involves the upper limbs, the patient will complain of "clumsiness," reporting activity such as dropping cups or plates or spilling liquids when surprised or when laughing. These attacks are short and do not resemble the "classic" full-blown attack of cataplexy. They are often ignored by physicians, despite being by far the most common form of attack. Without an electromyographic recording, their shortness may not make them obvious, even to a skilled clinician. The duration of each cataplectic attack—partial or total—is highly variable. They usually range from a few seconds to two minutes and rarely up to 30 minutes. Attacks can be elicited by emotion, stress, fatigue, or heavy meals. Laughter and anger seem to be the most common triggers, but the attacks can also be induced by a feeling of elation when listening to music, reading a book, or watching a movie. Cataplexy may be induced merely by remembering a happy or funny situation, and it may also occur without clear precipitating acts or emotions.

Cataplexy is associated with an inhibition of monosynaptic H-reflexes and of the multisynaptic tendon reflexes. H-reflex activity is fully suppressed physiologically only during REM sleep, which emphasizes the relationship between the motor inhibition of REM sleep and the sudden atonia and areflexia seen during a cataplectic attack.

Sleep paralysis is a terrifying experience that occurs in the narcoleptic when falling asleep or awakening. Patients find themselves suddenly unable to move the limbs, to speak, or even to breathe deeply. This state is frequently accompanied by hallucinations. During an episode of sleep paralysis, the patient is powerless to move the extremities, to speak, or to open the eyes, although he or she is fully aware of the condition and able to recall it completely afterward. In most episodes of sleep paralysis, but especially the first occurrence, the patient will experience extreme anxiety, such as that associated with the fear of dying. With more experience of the phenomenon, however, the patient usually learns that episodes are brief and benign, rarely lasting longer than a few minutes and always end spontaneously. The anxiety is often greatly intensified by the terrifying hallucinations that may accompany the sleep paralysis.

Sleep onset in the narcoleptic patient, either during daytime sleep episodes or at night, may be unpleasant with vivid hypnagogic hallucinations. These hallucinations are often visual, usually consisting of simple forms (colored circles, parts of objects, and so forth) that are constant or change in size. The image of an animal or a person may present itself abruptly in black and white, or more often in color. Auditory hallucinations are also common, although other senses are seldom involved. The auditory hallucinations can range from a collection of sounds to an elaborate melody. The patient may also be menaced by threatening sentences or harsh invectives. Another common and interesting type of hallucination reported at sleep onset involves elementary cenesthopathic feelings (i.e., experiencing picking, rubbing, or light touching), changes in location of body parts (arm or leg), or feelings of levitation or extracorporeal experiences (moving the body in space or floating above the bed) that may be quite elaborate. (For example, the patient may report, "I am above my bed, and I can also see my body below, or I am a few feet up, and people jump over my body.") The association with sleep paralysis has led researchers to postulate gamma loop involvement in some of these hallucinations. The abrupt motor inhibition that involves the spinal cord motorneurons may lead to a significant decrease in the feedback of information normally used by the central nervous system (CNS) to gauge the position of the body and the relation of the limb segments to each other. Night sleep is often interrupted by repeated awakenings and sometimes accompanied by terrifying dreams.

The first symptoms of narcolepsy often develop near puberty. The peak age at which reported symptoms occur is between 15 and 25 years of age, but narcolepsy and other symptoms have been noted at five or six years of age; a second, smaller peak of onset has been noted between 35 and 45 years, near menopause in women. EDS and irresistible sleep episodes usually occur as the first symptoms, either independently or associated with one or more other symptoms. They are enhanced by high environmental temperature, indoor activity, and idleness. Symptoms may abate with time, but they never phase out completely. Attacks of cataplexy generally appear in conjunction with abnormal episodes of sleep but may occur as much as 20 years later. They occasionally, but seldom, occur before the abnormal sleepiness, in which case they are a major source of difficulty in diagnosis. They can vary in frequency from a few episodes during the subject's entire lifetime to one or several episodes per day. Hypnagogic hallucinations and sleep paralysis do not affect all subjects and are often transitory. Disturbed nocturnal sleep seldom occurs in the first stages and generally builds up with age. Narcolepsy leads to a variety of complications, such as driving or machine-related accidents and difficulties at work. Without question, narcolepsy can responsible for disability, forced retirement, or job dismissal, even from relatively low-level jobs. Impotence and depression are common complications.

There is controversy concerning the criteria needed to confirm the diagnosis of narcolepsy. Japanese clinicians and researchers have indicated in the past that their American counterparts have given too much credence to polygraphic (sleep study) criteria and the presence of two or more sleep-onset REM periods on the Multiple Sleep Latency Test (MSLT). In Japan, a positive history of cataplexy associated with EDS is systematically required for the diagnosis of narcolepsy. Undoubtedly, the presence of cataplexy is pathognomonic of narcolepsy, but it may be difficult to rely on this criterion alone, particularly when cataplexy is partial—that is, limited to the head and neck or neck and upper arms.

2.2. CNS Hypersomnia

CNS hypersomnia is another condition of excessive daytime sleepiness, characterized by recurrent daytime sleepiness but without the abrupt sleep attacks or cataplexy seen in narcolepsy. The daytime sleepiness is isolated. Historically, this syndrome has had a number of labels, including essential narcolepsy, independent narcolepsy, nonrapid eye movement (NREM) sleep narcolepsy, idiopathic hypersomnia, functional hypersomnia, and harmonious hypersomnia. It is important to differentiate clearly CNS hypersomnia from the narcolepsy syndrome and from the daytime sleepiness related to self-induced sleep deprivation and nocturnal sleep disturbances (i.e., sleep apnea or periodic leg movement syndrome). However, the distinction from the narcolepsy syndrome can be difficult because the two disorders have many similarities, including age of symptom onset, nonremission of symptoms over the lifespan, and a hetero-familial tendency. The upper airway resistance syndrome may be another difficult differential diagnosis. Finally, several etiological factors may be responsible for the isolated daytime somnolence seen in idiopathic CNS hypersomnia syndrome, which renders definitive diagnosis and treatment more difficult.

3. GENETICS OF NARCOLEPSY

The investigation of the genetics of narcolepsy was greatly advanced when it was reported that 100% of the studied Japanese narcoleptic patients presented a class II antigen of the major histocompatibility complex known at that time as DR2. British, French, Canadian, and U.S. investigators confirmed that the great majority of studied Caucasian narcoleptics were also DR2 DQw1 Dw2 positive. Progress in the typology of class II antigens led to the creation of a new nomenclature in 1990, and the term DR15 DQw6 DW2 has replaced DR2.

It was demonstrated in 1989 that DR2 DQwl was neither sufficient nor necessary for the development of narcolepsy in both independent and familial cases. Nonetheless, investigations involving different clinics have emphasized the importance of DQw1 (DQw6 under the new World Health Organization [WHO] HLA nosology) as the best current HLA marker for narcolepsy. Only 70% of African-American narcoleptics, for example, carry DR2 (DRwl5 under new nosology) but nearly all carry the DQw1 (DWw6) subtype. The HLA DR and DQ molecules are heterodimers formed by the association of an alpha and a beta chain. These chains are encoded by specific genes. In Caucasian and Japanese subjects, the DQBeta1-0602 gene (located on the DQw6) is the best HLA marker for narcolepsy. However, authentic cases of narcolepsy with cataplexy do exist that are negative for DQBeta1-0602, which affirms the existence of the involvement of another gene in determining narcolepsy.

A greater understanding of the genetics and pathophysiology of narcolepsy has been possible through the discovery of the disease in animals such as dogs and horses. This has allowed for the development of an animal model for research. A canine model of the disease is available in which an autosomal recessive gene has been identified. The canine narcolepsy gene, *canarc*, plays a role in the immune system. It is involved in immunoglobulin class switching, which for example, allows an IgM molecule to change to IgG. This has lead to a search for immunopathological mechanism for the disease. To date, no such mechanism has been identified. Narcolepsy patients do not have the expected serological markers of a typical autoimmune disease. Of interest, the immuné-modulator thalidomide can induce narcolepsy.

The differential diagnosis of hypersomnia is broad, and includes:

- Narcolepsy
- Idiopathic and post-traumatic hypersomnia
- Obstructive sleep apnea syndrome
- Upper airway resistance syndrome
- Sleep restriction (insufficient total sleep time; sleep deprivation)
- Circadian phase delays or advances resulting in sleep restriction
- Depression; certain medical, endocrinological and neurological conditions; chronic fatigue syndrome
- Primary disorders of sleep such as nocturnal myoclonus

One can conclude that the current evidence supports the hypothesis that transmission of narcolepsy is multifactorial and involve at least two genes, one of which is non-HLA related. Investigation of monozygotic twins discordant for narcolepsy also strongly supports the idea that environmental factors have a critical role in the development of narcolepsy. Unfortunately, funding for narcolepsy research is relatively scarce, a result of a lack of awareness among physicians and the general public of the impact of narcolepsy.

4. DIFFERENTIAL DIAGNOSIS OF HYPERSOMNOLENCE

There are several entities that need to be well differentiated in patients with excessive daytime sleepiness (EDS). Narcolepsy is a common diagnostic consideration, but it is not the most difficult. When the patient has EDS, a positive history of cataplexy, and the presence of two or more sleep-onset REM periods on the MSLT, there is little difficulty diagnosing narcolepsy. However, narcolepsy may initially present as isolated EDS, and the positive diagnosis may be in doubt for months or even years. Considering the importance of proper diagnosis for epidemiological and genetic studies, it is better to classify the disorder as "idiopathic hypersomnia" until the cataplexy develops. Neither HLA typing nor sleep onset REM periods are necessarily pathognomonic.

Cataplectic attacks may be confused with seizures; in particular, atonic seizures or drop attacks might be diagnosed instead of cataplexy, which would obviously result in inappropriate therapy. The main distinguishing feature is the retention of consciousness in an attack of cataplexy. The patient should not be amnestic during brief episodes of cataplexy; however, vertebrobasilar insufficiency producing ischemia in the ventral pons and medulla can be a difficult condition to distinguish on this basis alone. In this case, the age of the patient and a history of vascular disease usually help. The complaint of sleepiness and the positive MSLT findings may also be similar in patients with significant daytime sleepiness as a sequel of severe head trauma. The past medical history, which often includes an initial coma after the head trauma, is enlightening in these cases. The daytime somnolence seen in association with communicating hydrocephalus of unknown etiology also does not differ clinically from CNS hypersomnia. Imaging of the brain, which confirms the hydrocephalus, distinguishes this syndrome from idiopathic CNS hypersomnia. A careful history will differentiate these patients from those with chronic insufficient nocturnal sleep who also have daytime sleepiness.

Obstructive sleep apnea (OSA) syndrome might also be misdiagnosed as narcolepsy. The term "narcolepsy" has been used in medicine for many more years than has OSA. Narcolepsy was often used to describe any form of unexplained hypersomnolence. This is why patients with obstructive sleep apnea may report having older relatives diagnosed with "narcolepsy." Both are chronic conditions with decreased alertness. However, patients with narcolepsy will report that brief naps are refreshing, whereas patients with OSA may feel worse after a nap. Cataplexy is only found in narcoleptics. The clinician must keep in mind that obstructive sleep apnea is more common with advancing age. Therefore, an older narcoleptic patient could have worsening daytime alertness as a result of the development of OSA. Typically, the degree of excessive daytime sleepiness is not progressive in aging with narcolepsy. For unknown reasons, the comorbidity of narcolepsy and obstructive sleep apnea is higher than predicted by their prevalence.

4.1. Upper Airway Resistance Syndrome

Idiopathic CNS hypersomnia must above all be distinguished from upper airway resistance syndrome (UARS). Patients with UARS complain of isolated EDS. However, interviews frequently indicate that the patient snores during sleep. A prospective study performed in a sleep clinic reported snoring in 100% of the men but an absence of snoring in 25% of the women with the syndrome.

Examinations of these subjects often reveal a triangular face or a steep mandibular plane, a highly arched palate, a class II malocclusion, and a retroposition of the mandible. The patients are usually nonobese. Cephalometric x-rays have indicated the presence of a small space behind the base of the tongue (posterior airway space), often near the location of the hyoid bone.

Patients with UARS present repetitive short (transient) alpha electroencephalographic arousals lasting three to fourteen seconds that regularly interrupt snoring periods. Standard polygraphic recordings of these subjects suggest the diagnosis on the basis of the presence of these repetitive transient arousals and increases in snoring just before the arousal. Increase in inspiratory time and decrease in expiratory time may be found with well-calibrated sensors. No significant change in arterial oxygen saturation is usually seen, and the respiratory disturbance index is low (<5).

Once the diagnosis has been suggested, it must be confirmed. Confirmation requires a referral to a sleep disorders specialist. Polygraphic monitoring with a small caliber esophageal catheter or balloon, a face mask, and a pneumotachygraph will demonstrate decreases (increasing negative pressure) in intrapleural (endoesophageal) pressure with each breath just before each arousal. One to three breaths later there maybe a decrease in airflow and tidal volume. Clinical investigation may not require use of a face mask and pneumotachygraph; however, measurement of intrapleural (endoesophageal) pressure, an indicator of respiratory effort, is needed. The tidal volume could drop in the one to three breaths just preceding the transient arousal. In contrast with obstructive sleep apnea syndrome, no complete obstruction occurs. A transient decrease in flow precedes and triggers the arousal, but the tidal volume decrease is so transient that pulse oximetry is not significantly affected. The sleep fragmentation occurring with this syndrome is one of the factors leading to the EDS complaint. The complex diagnostic procedure described can demonstrate the upper airway's resistance, but it also disturbs sleep significantly. The diagnosis can then be confirmed by way of use of nasal continuous positive airway pressure as a therapeutic test. The proper prescribed positive end-expiratory pressure of the nasal continuous positive airway pressure equipment is determined during polysomnography on the basis of snoring and esophageal pressure measurements. A repeat evaluation during continuous positive airway pressure treatment one month later should demonstrate improvement when compared with baseline. It is critical that this syndrome be excluded before idiopathic CNS hypersomnia is diagnosed.

5. EVALUATION AND WORK-UP

After a thorough history and physical examination, three tests have been designed to evaluate sleepiness objectively: electronic pupillogram; Multiple Sleep Latency Test (MSLT), and continuous 24- or 36-hour polysomnographic monitoring.

5.1. Electronic Pupillogram

The electronic pupillogram is a method of measuring decreased levels of sleepiness. The technique is based on the fact that peripheral autonomic manifestations are associated with states of arousal-excitation as well as with sleep. The size of the pupil is an index of autonomic activity. It was demonstrated conclusively that the pupil constricts during sleep. A normal alert individual sitting quietly in total darkness can maintain a stable pupil diameter, usually well above 7 mm, for at least 10 minutes, without subjective difficulty or pupillary oscillation. Often, this technique is performed with a series of light stimuli. The pupillary diameter in excessively sleepy patients is unstable when they are adapting to the dark. There are problems and limitations with this technique. Patients with ocular problems or autonomic CNS lesions must be identified and excluded. A patient's ability and willingness to cooperate are critical. Excessively sleepy subjects have trouble avoiding lid-drooping or closure. Small initial pupil diameters, dark irises, and excessive eye makeup all pose problems. Finally, the data may be difficult to interpret, particularly if recording conditions are not excellent and standardized. Although at one time experts did attempt to use pupillography to diagnose narcolepsy, it essentially diagnoses only sleepiness. This test does not indicate the underlying causes of EDS.

5.2. MSLT

The MSLT was designed by Carskadon and Dement to measure physiological sleep tendencies in the absence of alerting factors. It consists of four to six scheduled naps or trials, usually at 0900, 1100, 1300, 1500, and 1700 hours, during which the subject is polygraphically monitored in a comfortable, soundproof, dark bedroom. The latency between lights-out time and sleep onset is calculated for each nap. The type of sleep, REM or non-REM, is also noted. After each 20-min monitoring period, patients must stay awake until the following scheduled trial. The MSLT records the latency for each nap, the mean sleep latency, and the presence or absence of REM sleep in any of the naps. On the basis of polygraphic recording, REM sleep that occurs within 15 min of sleep onset is considered a sleep-onset REM period.

In normal populations, MSLT scores vary with age, puberty being the critical landmark, with prepubertal children between the ages of six and eleven years appearing hyperalert. In adults, mean MSLT scores under eight minutes are generally considered to be in the pathological range; those over ten minutes are considered normal. When the range is between eight and ten minutes, age factors interact, so the test

---

The Multiple Sleep Latency Test (MSLT) is the cornerstone of the diagnosis of hypersomnolence and of narcolepsy:

- The rapidity with which the patient is able to fall asleep is a quantitative measure of sleepiness.
- The sleep stage which occurs in these brief daytime naps indicates the "REM propensity."
- Both pathologic sleepiness and REM propensity are reasonably well-defined in certain populations, including narcolepsy.

---

must be interpreted with greater care; mean scores of eight to ten minutes represent a gray zone.

An MSLT performed alone with no overnight sleep study has the same drawbacks as pupillography does; that is, it measures sleepiness regardless of its cause, which may be simply sleep deprivation. The MSLT also ignores repetitive microsleeps that can lead, in borderline cases, to daytime impairment not scored by conventional analysis. To be clinically relevant, the test must be conducted under specific conditions. Subjects must have abstained from medication for a sufficient period (usually 15 days) so that drug effect and drug withdrawal effect are avoided. On the basis of sleep diaries, their sleep-wake schedules are stabilized. On the night preceding the MSLT, they undergo a nocturnal polysomnogram—that is, a polygraphic recording of variables defining sleep states and stages, waking (electroencephalogram, electro-oculogram, chin electromyogram), and other biological variables (cardiac, pulmonary, gastrointestinal, and so on). Throughout the total nocturnal sleep period, any sleep-related biological abnormalities responsible for sleep fragmentation and sleep deprivation are recorded.

The nocturnal polysomnogram indicates the underlying cause for the complaint of sleepiness; the MSLT indicates the severity of the problem. Once the nocturnal sleep recording has eliminated specific diseases and demonstrated that a patient is sleeping normally during the night, the MSLT confirms the diagnosis of narcolepsy with the presence of two or more sleep-onset REM periods.

It was proposed adding a test for the maintenance of wakefulness to the MSLT in order to measure the patient's ability not to fall asleep, but to maintain wakefulness. This test involves the patient being instructed to remain awake in a comfortable sitting position in a dark room for five trials similar to the MSLT. The test may be helpful in specific pharmacological trials, but it has proved unsatisfactory as a diagnostic procedure.

5.3. Continuous 24- or 36-Hour Polysomnographic Monitoring

Another procedure has been a continuous 24- or 36-hour polysomnographic monitoring that provides information about the actual number, duration, times, and types of daytime sleep episodes, as well as the disrupted night sleep. In addition, this long polygraphic recording may identify the dissociated REM sleep inhibitory process characterizing cataplexy with an awake electroencephalogram and electro-oculogram recording associated with elimination of chin and muscle twitches that are typical of REM sleep. Broughton and colleagues have proposed using auditory-evoked potentials in the evaluation of sleepiness; but, once again, this test, which may be helpful in evaluating pharmacological agents, has not been sufficiently discriminative to be used as a diagnostic tool.

6. DIAGNOSTIC CRITERIA FOR NARCOLEPSY

As mentioned previously, there is currently controversy concerning the criteria needed to affirm narcolepsy. A mean sleep latency of less than five minutes and two sleep-onset REM episodes on an MSLT are the minimum criteria for narcolepsy if there is no other explanation for excessive daytime sleepiness. In Japan, a positive history of cataplexy associated with EDS is systematically required for the diagnosis of narcolepsy. Undoubtedly, the presence of cataplexy is pathognomonic of narcolepsy, but it may be difficult to rely on this criterion alone, particularly when cataplexy is subtle. Some experts have recommended caution before the diagnosis of narcolepsy is given, even if sleepiness and two or more sleep-onset REM periods at MSLT are present. A study found that only 84% of the individuals with complaints of EDS and documentation of cataplexy have two or more sleep-onset REM periods at MSLT. These data indicate that false positives and negatives can be found with a single 24-hour polygraphic investigation. It has been recommended that "narcolepsy" be used only when EDS and at least a positive history of cataplexy are associated with two or more sleep onset REM periods. If a history of cataplexy is absent, a more descriptive term such as "EDS with several sleep-onset REM periods" should be used. The requirement of a positive history of cataplexy would eliminate subjects in the developing phase of the syndrome that can take several years. However, the use of strict criteria will allow better epidemiological studies.

7. REFERRAL AND TREATMENT CONSIDERATIONS

Patients with suspected narcolepsy should be evaluated by a physician with expertise in sleep disorders. It is very important to make an accurate diagnosis, because patients will need a lifetime of treatment with controlled substances. The clinician must be aware of the possibility of malingering to obtain amphetamines. Diagnostic evaluations are ideally carried out in sleep disorders clinics accredited by the American Sleep Disorders Association (ASDA). Once a definitive diagnosis has been established and effective therapy has begun, the patient can continue to be treated by the primary care physicians. The sleep specialist would then act as a consultant when needed. Patients with narcolepsy may require frequent office visits owing to legal limitations placed on the prescription of stimulant medication. Primary care physicians also need to monitor for the development of hypertension, abnormal liver function, depression, irritability, anorexia, insomnia, or psychosis associated with the treatment medications.

The goal of all therapeutic approaches in narcolepsy is to control the narcoleptic symptoms and to allow the patient to continue full participation in familial and professional daily activities. However, drug prescriptions must take into account possible side effects, keeping in mind the fact that narcolepsy is a lifelong illness, and patients will have to receive medication for years. Tolerance or addiction may be seen with some compounds. Treatment of narcolepsy thus balances avoidance of secondary side effects and tolerance, with maintenance of an active life. Clinicians are not unanimous on the end points of therapeutic success, drug dosages, or acceptability of unwanted effects. In addition, patients vary widely in their assessment of the goals of therapy and acceptability of side effects. Some clinicians believe that the aim of therapy is not for patients to be awake and alert all day, but for them to be awake and alert only when they need to be awake and alert. Other clinicians believe that the patients should optimally be alert all day; when patients are on proper treatment, they will not require naps; and they will accept a certain level of side effects to reach this goal. There may be a huge difference in what side effects are acceptable to the physicians and what side effects are acceptable to the patients. On one hand, some patients might not accept even mild tremor, even though they may be much more alert with even small doses of stimulants, whereas other patients readily accept tremor, fidgety behavior, irritability, and nocturnal insomnia as the price they pay to maintain alertness all day. The physician might not accept elevation of the blood pressure as a side effect, even though the patient would probably be unaware of this effect.

Because of the differences in end points, there are differences in the approach to use of medications. Thus, some clinicians seldom, if ever, exceed the usual dosage ranges, whereas others believe that the dosage that is acceptable for an individual patient is whatever is required to make that patient alert all day. With the latter approach, some patients are prescribed much larger than the usual dosages of stimulants. Thus, because of the marked interpatient variability in response to a dosage of a stimulant and because of differences in therapeutic goals, the actual dosages used in clinical practice can vary widely.

As a general rule, avoidance of amphetamines is recommended during pregnancy. However, the little data available do not indicate obvious increased fetal risk or teratogenicity. One must acknowledge that first trimester of pregnancy is often associated the development of sleepiness in normal women, and this may become an intolerable burden for a narcoleptic. If medication must be used, the short half-life methylphenidate makes it desirable for this case.

Future research should include the establishment of a pharmacovigilance database as is used, for example, in specific drugs administered to certain cardiac patients or cancer patients. This database could help resolve the uncertainty that exists concerning the appropriateness of specific dosages and the relationship between blood levels and side effects or tolerance. Treatment for each patient could be better individualized, and dosages that always have to be adjusted on the basis of a good patient-physician exchange would be obtained with a clearer rationale. Such a database would also provide information to patients on the long-term risks of their treatment.

The current lack of complete knowledge of these factors helps explain the large differences in prescription patterns. For example, a survey with more than 1000 narcoleptic patients revealed that many of them were being prescribed very low dosages of medications, whereas a surprisingly large number of patients were being prescribed dosages in excess of the highest recommended dosage. For the three most commonly used medications—methylphenidate, dextroamphetamine, and pemoline—at least 10% of patients were at or above the highest manufacturer recommended dosage. The physician and the patient must always remember that the long-term ramifications of using such high dosages of medications for a lifelong illness are unknown.

The drug treatments recommended in Table 2 reflect our current clinical practice at the Stanford University Sleep Disorders Clinic that are based on our own patient surveys, reviews of literature, and patient-physician interaction. We believe that these recommendations form a reasonable guideline for the treatment of most patients with narcolepsy.

Table 2
Drugs for Narcolepsy Currently Available

Treatment of excessive daytime sleepiness

Stimulants
    5–60 mg/d Dextroamphetamine
    20–25 mg/d Methamphetamine[a]
    10–60 mg/d Methylphenidate
    4–8 mg/d (divided dosage) Mazindol
    37.5 mg/d Pemoline
Adjunct-effect drugs (i.e., improve EDS taken with stimulant)
    2.5–10 mg/d Protriptyline
    50–200 mg/d Viloxazine

Treatment of auxiliary symptoms (e.g., cataplexy)

Antidepressants (with atropinic side effects)
    2.5–20 mg/d Protriptyline
    25–200 mg/d Imipramine
    25–200 mg/d Clomipramine
    25–200 mg/d Desipramine
Antidepressants (without atropinic side effects)
    50–200 mg/d Viloxazine
    20–60 mg/d Fluoxetine

Experimental drugs (available in some countries)

Stimulants
    Modafinil
    Codeine (given as stimulant)
Cataplexy antagonist and mild stimulant
    γ-Hydroxybutyrate[b]

[a]Occasionally, depending on clinical response, the dose may be outside the usual dosage range.
[b]Not available in many parts of the world and the United States.

The drugs most widely used to treat EDS are the CNS stimulants. Amphetamines were first proposed in 1935. The alerting effect of a single oral dose of amphetamine is at its maximum two to four hours after administration, and many patients require a single daily or twice-daily dose. However, a number of side effects may arise that include irritability, tachycardia, nocturnal sleep disturbances, and sometimes tolerance and drug dependence. The use of methylphenidate was later encouraged, because of faster action and lower incidence of side effects. Pemoline, an oxazolidine derivative with a longer half-life and a slower onset of action, is less efficient but well tolerated. When medications are

> The treatment of narcolepsy generally involves a two-pronged approach:
>
> - Treatment of hypersomnolence with CNS stimulants
> - Treatment of cataplexy, sleep paralysis or hypnogogic hallucinations with anti-depressants, especially the tricyclic compounds

initiated, pemoline is typically the first stimulant tried. Modafinil, a stimulant medication available in France, has been reported to bring substantial improvement. Modafinil has received a "go ahead" from the FDA for sale in the United States in the near future. This agent, 2-[(diphenylmethyl)sulfinyl] acetamide, is distinct from other CNS stimulants in its chemical and pharmacologic properties. It enhances alertness, but is less active in the dopaminergic brain systems, and does not increase locomotor activity in animals as much as amphetamines and methylphenidate. There also appears to be less abuse potential. The exact mechanism of action is uncertain. Effective doses are in the 200–400 mg range, given once daily. Modafinil is associated with headaches with increasing dosage. Mazindol, an imidazoline derivative, has been shown to reduce the number of daytime sleep episodes in narcoleptics in a dose range of 3–6 mg. Propranolol may be effective but requires large doses. Gamma-hydroxybutyrate, given orally at bedtime and at the time of a night awakening may be of value, but its efficacy varies among patients. It is available in France and Canada and is being investigated in the US; the full evaluation of γ-hydroxybutyrate is incomplete.

The treatment of cataplexy, sleep paralysis, and hypnagogic hallucinations involves tricyclic medications. Clomipramine has been widely used with good responses. Other tricyclic medications, such as protriptyline, imipramine, and desipramine, are also effective; however, the atropinic side effects, particularly impotence in men, have led to the search for new compounds. Clonidine, a potent REM sleep suppressant, is not a first-line drug, because of too many side effects. Viloxazine hydrochloride, an norepinephrine (NE) reuptake blocker that seems well tolerated by patients, including the elderly, is one of these new compounds, but is not available in the US. A progressive dosage increase of viloxazine hydrochloride from 100 to 200 to 300 mg daily may completely avoid the appearance, in rare cases, of headaches or nausea in elderly subjects. Fluoxetine has also been reported to be helpful against cataplexy, and other selective serotonin reuptake inhibitors, such as paroxetine, are worthy of trial in necessary cases. Although animal data suggest that selective increase in serotonin levels by these agents might not help cataplexy, but the data in humans are quite limited. Monoamine oxidase inhibitors, such as phenelzine, have been used to treat patients with intractable narcolepsy-cataplexy, but the frequent dangerous side effects have severely limited their usage, especially if they must be combined with stimulants. Selegiline, the new monoamine oxidase inhibitor, has less of the tyramine-related side effects and appears to be helpful in the treatment of EDS. The pharmacological activity of the drug on sleepiness may be related to levamphetamine, a metabolite, may explain its efficacy. Although yohimbine has been shown to be effective against canine narcolepsy, it has little effect in human cataplexy.

A comparison of the efficacy of putative therapeutic agents on daytime sleepiness as measured by the MSLT has been published. The authors normalized the data obtained from 179 narcoleptic subjects, reporting the results as a percentage of normal values obtained from a control group. The drugs tested were dextroamphetamine, methylphenidate, pemoline, modafinil (CRL), protriptyline, viloxazine, ritanserin, codeine, and γ-hydroxybutyrate. The study shows that even at the highest recommended dosage, no drug brings narcoleptics to a normal alertness. Dextroamphetamine and methylphenidate improved patients' alertness the most; γ-hydroxybutyrate, protriptyline, and ritanserin had a nonsignificant impact; viloxazine, modafinil, and pemoline had a mild to moderate impact; however, no objective comparisons of different drugs on the same subjects was ever performed.

Cataplexy, sleep paralysis, and hypnagogic hallucinations are best treated by noradrenergic reuptake blockers. Most tricyclic antidepressants have noradrenergic reuptake-blocking properties, but they often have other properties that may lead to side effects. Clomipramine has long been the treatment of choice in Europe for auxiliary symptoms, in dosages from 75–150 mg/d. It is now available in the US. Imipramine (75–150 mg), desipramine, and protriptyline (5–15 mg) are also effective. Fluoxetine can help cataplexy with somewhat less efficacy than the other medications, probably more through its mild NE reuptake-blocking properties than through its strong serotonergic reaction.

Nocturnal sleep disturbances seem to be better controlled by γ-hydroxybutyrate than by the benzodiazepines. The advantage of improving nocturnal sleep is significant, not only for daytime sleepiness, but also for cataplexy. However, stimulant medications will often be necessary with γ-hydroxybutyrate. Patients who present with all the clinical symptoms of narcolepsy will frequently need a combination of drugs, particularly stimulants and tricyclics; γ-hydroxybutyrate or a benzodiazepine may sometimes be added at night.

The nocturnal sleep disturbances of narcolepsy may be related to muscle twitches and periodic leg movements. Muscle twitches may be part of narcolepsy, but it may also be a complication of large doses of tricyclic medications. If a patient abruptly complains of an abnormal amount of muscle jerks, a decrease in tricyclic intake may be the solution. However, in most cases the jerks are not related to drug intake. L-Dopa with a dopa decarboxylase inhibitor (Sinemet 10–100, containing 10 mg carbidopa and 100 mg levodopa) may be helpful. This drug must be taken at bedtime, although its short duration of action may require a second dose in the middle of the night. Benzodiazepines may also be helpful.

Two other therapeutic approaches must be emphasized: short daytime naps and patient support groups. A 15–20 min nap taken three times daily will help maintain a satisfactory level of vigilance. Naps may have to be repeated throughout the day, because the "refractory" sleep period after a nap will oscillate between 90 and 120 min. Undoubtedly, narcolepsy is a disabling disorder leading, in many instances, to loss of gainful employment because of daytime sleepiness and automatic behavior. It is also a disorder often poorly understood by patients, family members, and peers that can result in rejection from families and other social entities, in divorces, in loss of self-esteem, and in depressive reactions. For these reasons, and in consideration of age of onset, it is important to put narcoleptic patients in contact with support groups and to help with the creation of regional narcolepsy associations and patient groups.

The aim of narcolepsy treatment is to maintain the patient's wakefulness and alertness throughout the day. However, the medications currently available (mainly amphetamines) often have significant side effects, and treatment plans must therefore be tailored to individual preference and tolerance; there must also be good communication between the physician and the patient. Often, complete alertness throughout the day is not achievable despite medications.

Many European countries have banned amphetamines because of their side effects and the potential for abuse. It is also in these countries that all new stimulant drugs currently under experimental trial have been discovered. There are patients who have now taken amphetamines for 30–40 years without ill effects. Many authors have described the effects of amphetamines. In 1973, Dement and Guilleminault reported on a paradoxical effect of amphetamines in narcoleptics and hypersomniacs; increased sleepiness was found in 33 subjects at the dose of 100 mg/d or more. This effect disappeared with reduction of the daily dose.

Whereas abnormal involuntary movements including repetitive complex volitional movements have been described in amphetamine addicts, abnormal movements have never been observed in our narcoleptic patients and seem to be undescribed in the literature. More common is a light tremor of the fingers; this was noted in 8% of subjects taking large doses of amphetamines. David Parkes reported that response to amphetamines varies with different subjects. In their study, similar blood levels of amphetamines were achieved in both good and poor responders. Age of onset of narcolepsy and frequency and duration of narcoleptic attacks did not seem to be important variables. Also, one third of the patients rapidly became tolerant of amphetamines and needed to double their dosage to obtain some control of symptoms. The reasons for this variation between patients in development of tolerance are poorly understood.

The plasma elimination rate for amphetamines is increased in dependent versus drug-naive subjects. With long-term treatment, an increased drug affinity for tissues also seems to occur. The result of long-term or high dosages of amphetamines on brain NE in humans is unknown. The only available data are from animal (predominantly rat) studies, which show depletion of presynaptic NE vesicles. The result of long-term amphetamine treatment on the fetus is also essentially unknown. A review of the teratogenicity of amphetamines in humans concluded that it was unlikely. In summary, this chapter indicates that although amphetamines are clearly related to certain side effects, there is wide variation between subjects with regard to response to medication, appropriate dosage level, and development of tolerance.

CASE STUDIES

Case 1

Becky is a nine-year-old girl who complains of being tired while spending the summer with her grandparents in Connecticut; she has been healthy her entire life. She now wants to sleep during the day. When playing soccer, she fell when she had a clear opportunity to score a goal. Her friends laughed at her because she slipped. She later confided to her mother that she knew she had not slipped and did not know why she fell. Later that summer, she started to have to look for something to lean on when she laughed. Her primary care physician ordered a workup for Lyme disease and later referred the patient to a neurologist.

DISCUSSION

Becky demonstrated many of features of narcolepsy; the most striking feature is the development of cataplexy when she fell prior to attempting to score a goal and weakness with laughter. The age of onset is younger than expected; in a prepubertal child with daytime sleepiness, myotonic dystrophy should be included in the differential diagnosis.

Case 2

James is a 21-year-old college student with a history of extreme anxiety with public speaking who complains of being tired during the day. He is taking sertraline for his anxiety prescribed by his primary care provider. His complaints of fatigue persist, and he reports occasional snoring, which leads to a referral to a sleep specialist. He reports sleeping about eight hours at night. He feels sleepy when driving long distances but has not gotten into any accidents. When he feels sleepy, a brief nap is refreshing; sometimes he will dream during a nap. There is some vague feeling of weakness in his jaw when he speaks in public. He denies cataplexy, hypnagogic hallucinations, and sleep paralysis. HLA typing, a nocturnal polysomnogram, and an MSLT were ordered. He agreed not to drive until a diagnosis and effective treatment were found. He was told to stop using the sertraline for three weeks prior to the sleep studies. His MSLT showed a mean sleep latency of three minutes with five sleep onset REM periods. No significant sleep apnea was present. The HLA typing was negative for expected narcolepsy markers. Urine toxicology screen was negative for common illegal street drugs. James is then started on stimulant medication, pemoline, and reports improved daytime function. Unfortunately, he later confides that he did not stop the sertraline until three days prior to his sleep study.

DISCUSSION

This true case demonstrates some of the complexity that can be found in practice. James is sleepy during the day, brief naps are refreshing, and he dreams during these brief naps. These are features narcolepsy, but they can also be seen in cases of inadequate sleep time or in sleep deprivation. The latter may be present in students. His vague jaw feelings may be a cataplexy equivalent. The initial sleep study results are characteristic of narcolepsy, but the sleep onset REM periods may be owing to abrupt medication withdrawal. Any medication that can suppress REM can have this effect when it is withdrawn. Medications to consider are tricyclic antidepressants, serotonin reuptake inhibitors, stimulants, and benzodiazepines. HLA typing be supportive of a diagnosis of narcolepsy, but it cannot currently be used to confirm or exclude the diagnosis unequivocally. Approximately 5–10% of narcoleptics will not have the expected HLA marker, and people with sleepiness for a different reason may be DQB10602 positive. Pemoline was started despite the diagnostic uncertainty, because the excessive sleepiness was severely affecting his daytime performance. The sleep studies were repeated during the summer school break when James was off all medications. The MSLT again showed a short sleep latency with five sleep-onset REM periods. A year later, James developed more clear-cut attacks of cataplexy.

SUGGESTED READINGS

Utlely M. *Narcolepsy: A Funny Disease that Is No Laughing Matter.* Self Published, Desoto, TX, 1995.

Kryger M, Roth T, Dement W. *Principles and Practice of Sleep Medicine.* W.B. Saunders, Philadelphia, 1994.

6   Obstructive Sleep Apnea Syndrome

Kingman P. Strohl

1. INTRODUCTION

Obstructive sleep apnea (OSA) and its sequela pose a significant health problem. People meeting minimal criteria for OSA treatment may comprise 2–4% of the general population, and there are pockets of increased prevalence, such as obese individuals and those with hypertension, myocardial infarction, or stroke. Sleep apnea also occurs in childhood; however, the prevalence is less well known.

The excessive daytime sleepiness that results from sleep apnea constitutes a personal risk as well as a societal risk, including motor vehicle accidents. Of individuals with the presenting symptom of disabling daytime sleepiness, obstructive sleep apnea is the leading medical cause.

OSA could contribute to the pathogenesis of other common diseases. One example is the coexistence of a critical lesion that produces angina

From: *Sleep Disorders: Diagnosis and Treatment*
Edited by: J. S. Poceta and M. M. Mitler © Humana Press Inc., Totowa, NJ

Table 1
Definition of Illness from OSA

A. Daytime sleepiness or other neurocognitive complaints associated with a significant degree of obstructive respiratory disturbances during sleep.
B. Reduction or elimination of symptoms with reduction or elimination of OSA.

and that of OSA; hence, the recognition and management of OSA is relevant to primary care practitioners. However, the diagnosis is made infrequently; one estimate is that recognized OSA is nearly 10-fold less than the prevalence in the community of moderately severe presentations of the illness.

Significant illnesses are likely to be caused by OSA if certain general conditions are met. Because a degree of apneic activity has been documented in normal populations who are free of sleep-related symptoms, one should distinguish "sleep-disordered breathing" from the clinical syndrome of OSA. The clinical syndrome not only has apneic activity during sleep, but also moderate to severe sleepiness during the day (or perhaps other symptoms, such as restless sleep). Also prominent among the conditions that should be met before ascribing a patient's symptoms to sleep-disordered breathing would be elimination of the symptoms after elimination of sleep apnea (Table 1).

2. CLINICAL PRESENTATIONS

The symptoms identified as associated with sleep apnea are listed in Table 2. These fall into three areas: daytime sleepiness, snoring and related symptoms, and "other." Excessive daytime sleepiness is present in as much as 30% of the general population, but much of this sleepiness results from a "voluntary" restriction of sleep. In fact, insufficient sleep time is so common that it can be considered quasi-normal in modern societies, albeit not recommended. There is a continuum of the severity of sleepiness, and disabling habitual sleepiness is accompanied by functional impairments such as an inability to drive an automobile, to work, or to maintain social functions. Sleep apnea is a major cause of disabling sleepiness and can exacerbate sleepiness caused by sleep restriction or shift work, for example. Some people might interpret sleepiness as fatigue or poor concentration, although usually the two can be distinguished by the patient and clinician with focused questioning. The neurocognitive complaints of OSA are thought to relate to the disturbed sleep produced by repetitive arousals from apneas.

Table 2
Some Presenting Symptoms of OSA

Sleepiness or fatigue (at least moderate severity)
Accidents or injury from sleep attacks
Habitual snoring
Apneas observed during sleep
Awakenings at night or restless sleep
Nocturnal angina[a]
Sentinel event: myocardial infarction, stroke[a]
Headache upon awakening[a]
Impotence[a]

[a]Uncommon as a sole presenting complaint.

Snoring is a hallmark symptom, but the likelihood of sleep apnea increases when there are clusters of additional symptoms or risk factors such as:

- Mandibular insufficiency, tonsillar hypertrophy, or other upper airway anomalies.
- Obesity or thick neck.
- Hypertension.
- Daytime sleepiness.
- Restlessness during sleep.

Snoring has been considered a hallmark symptom, however; it is not at all specific, since 50% of a general population will report that they snore. Instead, loud snoring that can be heard in the next room with snorts and pauses during sleep is far more suggestive of OSA. A colorful but apt term is "resuscitative snoring," which can often be described by the patient's bed partner quite accurately. This refers to the louder-than-usual snoring and snorting occurring after an apnea, when the patient has aroused him or herself. There is often movement of the body such as jerking of the arms or rolling over at this time.

Snoring is produced by turbulent airflow in the soft airway and is determined by many factors, some of which can change under certain circumstances or over time. Nasal resistance, the size of the upper airway, the compliance of the walls, and the characteristics of the inspiratory pressure generation all influence snoring. Because aspects of snoring (such as loudness) are the subjective impressions of a bedpartner, some skepticism is necessary when interpreting the history.

As stated, most patients who snore do not require evaluation for OSA, but there are also patients in whom severe sleep apnea can be present whose spouses are not aware of loud snoring, and even cases in which little snoring can be documented.

Less common presentations such nocturia, restlessness, awakening at night without cause, or with angina are less specific but possible presentations. Clusters of these symptoms increase the likelihood that the patient has OSA. For example, a person with nocturnal angina, resuscitative snores and daytime sleepiness has a high likelihood of OSA and would probably benefit from its recognition and treatment.

Community surveys with follow-up sleep studies emphasize that many persons have excess numbers of apneas without these symptoms. We do not know the clinical significance of these excessive numbers of apneas in asymptomatic individuals. It is possible that there are individual variations in sleepiness and in other consequences of apneic activity, some of which might change over time.

3. PHYSICAL EXAMINATION AND LABORATORY FINDINGS

There are few, if any, physical signs that definitively indicate the presence of sleep apnea. An estimated likelihood of apneic activity can be obtained from measurements of weight—in particular, body mass index (BMI). Obesity as a risk factor for sleep apnea is four times stronger than gender and two times stronger than age. Neck size (greater than 17 inches in males; greater than 15.5 inches in females) also has predictive value; at present, there are no specific measures other than weight and neck size that can be obtained on physical examination that correlate with airway size and function during sleep. Nonetheless, narrowed facies, retrognathia, and a high-arched palate have been described as being more common in patients with OSA. Pharyngeal abnormalities, such as markedly enlarged tonsils, when present in combination with symptoms of restless sleep and daytime sleepiness, indicate an increased likelihood of finding sleep apnea that might be managed surgically. Coexisting pulmonary and cardiac disease should be identified. A hypothyroid state should be ruled out (but only once). The routine measurement of arterial blood gases or pulmonary-function tests has not been found to be helpful in routine cases.

After the history and physical examination, one can estimate the potential impact of OSA on health status (*see* Subheading 6).

Obstructive sleep apnea produces:

• Acute desaturation and hypercapnia.
• Arousals from sleep and sympathetic nervous system activation.
• Long-term consequences of hypertension and sleepiness as a result of these nocturnal events.

4. ETIOLOGY AND PATHOPHYSIOLOGY

The site of obstruction in OSA is the posterior nasopharynx and oropharynx, down to the supraglottic area; the exact site of obstruction is not the same in all patients. There is an interaction of the bony structures at the base of the skull, the size and position of the mandible, and the soft structures of the pharynx that will determine the characteristics of an airway that might collapse during sleep. Among other things, these structures affect the size and position of the tongue, which forms the anterior portion of the supraglottic airway.

The current idea is that the onset of sleep is associated with a decrease in muscle activity that then permits passive closure of the pharyngeal airway, which is under the influence of negative pressure generated within the thorax. The immediate effect is a lack of airflow through the upper airway, with consequent hypercapnia (retention of CO_2) and oxyhemoglobin desaturation (fall in oxygen). Patients break from the apneas with a central nervous system arousal, usually a loud snort, accompanied by a surge in sympathetic nerve activity and blood pressure. The patient takes a few breaths and returns to sleep, only to repeat the process. The patient is usually not aware of this arousal, as it lasts only several seconds. The degree of desaturation can be mild in some patients, and dramatic in others—well below 60%—but the time course is brief, and resaturation usually occurs in less than 20 seconds or so. A particularly severe situation is when resaturation is not complete, thus lowering the overall mean SaO_2 for the night. Figure 1 shows a sleep laboratory example of repeated obstructive apneas with desaturation and arousal.

Long-term consequences of OSA appear to result from these intermittent arousals and hypoxic episodes. The most prominent are daytime sleepiness and systemic hypertension. The exact mechanism by which OSA produces daytime sleepiness is not certain, but the best correlation is between the degree of daytime sleepiness and the number of arousals during the night. Hypertension may be sustained, because of systemic catecholamine release overnight and/or up-regulation of the sympathetic nervous system and related to the arousals.

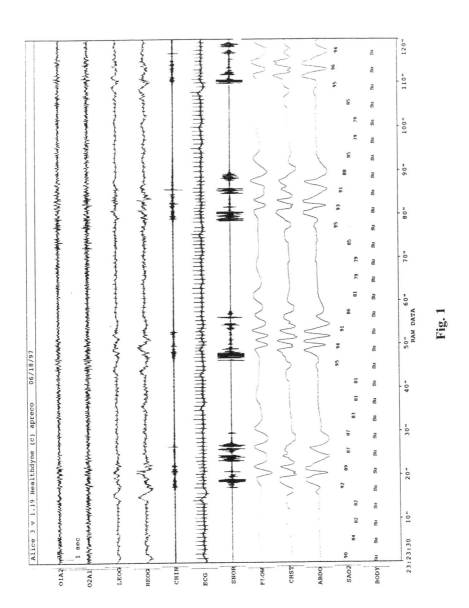

Fig. 1

122

- The diagnosis of Cheyne-Stokes respiration should be considered in patients with sleep complaints who have significant left ventricular dysfunction or cerebral vascular disease.
- Presenting symptoms can be either insomnia or daytime sleepiness.

5. CENTRAL SLEEP APNEA AND CHEYNE-STOKES RESPIRATION

There are different patterns of apnea found in clinical investigation and in sleep studies. The majority of persons with sleep apnea in the community have obstructive apneas in which there is a passive closure in the pharynx; hence, respiratory efforts are ineffective because of the closed upper airway. Central sleep apnea is a pattern in which there is a complete cessation of respiratory drive—that is, there are no respiratory efforts for some period of time. Different types and causes of central sleep apnea have been described; One common and important type is Cheyne-Stokes respiration (CSR), which is a series of waxing and waning respiratory efforts, with central apneas alternating with hyperpnea periods. CSR will be found in all healthy subjects that are acutely exposed to 10,000 to 14,000 feet elevation and is a product of the inherent instability of respiratory control. Central sleep apnea and CSR can be found in patients with congestive heart failure (CHF) or stroke; some present with daytime sleepiness, both with and without snoring. Insomnia may sometimes be the chief complaint of a patient with CHF and CSR. A sleep study is warranted in such patients who snore and are sleepy to exclude OSA.

The treatment of CSR is based on its impact on general health status and is sometimes approached differently from that of the more common OSA. For example, nasal oxygen is a commonly prescribed treatment

---

Fig. 1. *(previous page)* This example shows repeated obstructive apneas. The channels of this montage are labeled: Channels 1 and 2, EEG; 2 and 3, EPG; channel 4, chin surface EMG; channel 5, EKG; channel 6, snore detecting microphone taped on the neck; channel 7, airflow at the nose and mouth; channels 8 and 9, Respitrace bands; channel 10, saturation taken at the finger; and channel 11, body position (Su, supine). Note the cessation of airflow for 15 seconds followed by ineffective effort, then breakthrough snores, desaturation, and resaturation, and evidence of arousal on EEG, EMG, and heart rate. The patient is an overweight 45-year-old man with severe daytime sleepiness and bedpartner report of noisy, restless sleep.

for CSR in patients in whom OSA has been ruled out. Nasal oxygen can prevent the desaturations of CSR, and in some patients, blunt the hyperpneic phase and decrease arousals. Some research groups are evaluating the effect of nasal continuous positive airway pressure (CPAP) in CHF with and without CSR, but it is too early to make a general recommendation in this area.

6. WORKUP AND EVALUATION

A literature exists in the journals of family medicine, pediatrics, and internal medicine on the management of sleep apnea, but most of these articles provide details of specialist-based or center-based diagnosis and therapy. In part to address the need for materials directed at primary care practice, the National Center on Sleep Disorders Research has convened a panel of experts and primary care physicians to review the existing literature and make initial recommendations with regard to recognition of OSA. The NIH criteria for this type of document required a body of evidence upon which to make recommendations and applicability of recommendations to the broad range of practice settings and health systems in which physicians, nurses, and other health professionals will interact. None of these evaluation systems have been tested rigorously; however, there is a body of literature on the predictability of sleep apnea based on presenting signs and symptoms.

A scheme for the recognition is shown in Fig. 2. Questions like "Do you snore?" or "Are you sleepy?" are more helpful if they are answered negatively. If there is a positive response, more detailed questioning is usually needed to determine other potential functional correlates of sleep apneas. Those with the highest sensitivity are the functional correlates of excessive sleepiness. A common questionnaire used for assessment of sleepiness is the Epworth Sleepiness Scale (see Chapter 1). This eight-question survey, combined with a description of the character of the snoring, will permit an educated guess to the likelihood and the severity of OSA. Loud snorts and pauses during sleep occurring on a regular basis (i.e., five to seven times a week) is highly specific for the presence of apneic activity. Other features include family history of OSA and the presence or absence of cardiovascular risk factors, especially hypertension.

The association between sleep apnea and cardiovascular risk is clinically important, despite the fact that causal relationships have not been determined, nor are the mechanisms understood. For instance, studies from England have shown that patients in a primary practice setting with nocturnal angina have a higher likelihood of having OSA. Whether they

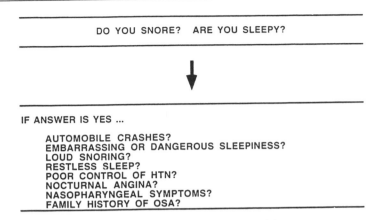

Fig. 2. Scheme for OSA recognition.

are also more likely to die in their sleep is not known, but effective treatment of OSA will eliminate nocturnal symptoms. Treatment of sleep apnea can reduce blood pressure into the "normal range" or make hypertension easier to control. However, at the present time, we know that treatment of blood pressure by medications can have beneficial effects on morbidity and mortality; similar information on the treatment of sleep apnea and this outcome are not available.

A detailed questionnaire of sleep habits can be useful. Such a questionnaire can be completed by the patient with the help of bed partners and other members of the family and will give the physician a reasonable idea of sleep-wake behavior, as well as breathing behavior during sleep. For example, the bedtime, wake-up times, and work schedules are critical to interpreting a complaint of sleepiness. The questionnaire can also assess other sleep-related symptoms such as restless legs syndrome, nocturnal cough or reflux, morning headaches, dreams, and confusion.

There is a spectrum in the severity of OSA (Table 3). Since OSA is a syndrome, there are no clear-cut agreed-upon measures of its severity. The standard numerical index of severity has been the number of apneas and hypopneas overnight per hour of sleep—that is, the Apnea-Hypopnea Index (AHI), alternatively called the Respiratory Disturbance Index. However, this measure, although significantly correlated with daytime sleepiness, by no means predicts all the variance in the syndrome. Similarly, one cannot rely only on the degree of oxyhemoglobin desaturation in making clinical decisions. Thus, the severity of OSA and the decisions for management are based on a composite of the clinical syndrome and the laboratory data. Those people with severe functional deficits and signs or symptoms of respiratory failure should

Table 3
Spectrum of Disease with OSA[a]

Reaction level	Signs and symptoms
Asymptomatic	Observed apneas or incidental finding of apneic activity[b]
Mild	Passive sleepiness with apneic activity and cardiovascular (CV) risk.
Moderate[c]	Active sleepiness, breathing-disturbed sleep, and CV risk.
Severe	Disabling sleepiness and cardiopulmonary failure, neurobehavioral deficits and increased apneic activity.

[a]Because of lack of a proven causal relationship between oxygen saturation indices (desaturation index, lowest oxygen saturation, time below 90%, and so on), arousal index, and MSLT with clinical outcome studies, this scale is based on clinical presentations and risk factors.
[b]Elevated age-adjusted AHI values.
[c]Controversy exists as to the distinct nature of those who have incomplete airway obstruction, do not meet some criteria for hypopneas during sleep, yet benefit from therapy ("high upper airway resistance syndrome").

be evaluated promptly by sleep studies, and therapy should be initiated as quickly as possible to restore ventilation during sleep. In those with moderate degrees of sleepiness in which the cause of the sleep disturbance is less clear, the primary care physician is in a position to counsel on sleep hygiene and the risks of driving and also to institute education on weight loss and to treat any concomitant medical conditions that might worsen gas exchange during the day. These concomitant conditions can include congestive heart failure, chronic obstructive lung disease, and nasal congestion and, would be treated by protocols directed at those problems.

In those individuals who snore but do not have sleepiness and in whom hypertension is easy to control with a single agent, conservative treatment can include the options listed in Table 4. If these fail, the primary care physician is in a position to provide information on the options to treat snoring with dental appliances, position therapy (i.e., placing a tennis ball in the back of the pajama shirt), or an external nasal dilators. These interventions for mild OSA and snoring are usually an out-of-pocket expense. Their costs relative to one another are listed in Table 5, but the benefits are less certain than the costs in any one individual. Success or failure can be determined primarily by the patient and his or her bedpartner.

If snoring persists and symptoms of sleepiness begin to arise, further evaluation may be indicated. There is a differential diagnosis for various aspects of OSA illness that appears to progress over time despite treatment or which presents *de novo* in a previously asymptomatic patient (Table 6).

Table 4
Conservative Measures to Reduce Simple Snoring

Treat hypothyroidism.
Treat nasal obstruction.
Diet/fitness to reduce neck size and abdominal girth.
Instruct the patient to avoid tobacco, alcohol, or medications that induce sleep
    such as sedatives, sleeping pills, and antihistamines.
Instruct the patient on measures to maximize sleep quality.

Table 5
Relative Cost for Relief of Simple Snoring for Six Months (Estimated)

Snore ball (tennis ball in a pocket sewn on the back of a nightshirt)	1
External nasal dilator	5
Mouthpiece fitted by dentist to reduce snoring	100
Uvulopalatal shaping (laser out-patient procedure)	250

Table 6
Differential Diagnosis of Sleep Complaints

Excessive daytime sleepiness
    Lifestyle, sleep restriction, restless legs syndrome, narcolepsy, drug use,
        head trauma or injury, other medical, psychiatric, or other sleep disorder.
Upper airway obstruction
    Neck mass, lymphoid enlargement (can be seen with early stages of HIV),
        nasal pharyngeal carcinoma, and brain stem tumor.

7. WHEN TO REFER

The primary care physician will determine, in conjunction with the patient, a threshold for referral. One might agree that one or more car accidents caused by sleepiness warrants an immediate referral, whereas less obvious sleepiness does not. An urgent workup is also indicated by the presence of nocturnal angina. It is clear that obesity itself, hypertension by itself, or snoring by itself does not necessarily indicate the need for rapid diagnosis and intervention. Also, it seems advisable to seek specialist advice before subjecting the patient to surgery (i.e., the laser-assisted uvuloplasty), even if only snoring (and not sleep apnea) is suspected.

As already emphasized, community studies have told us that there are wide ranges of apneic activity, as well as a wide range of symptomatic consequences. Given the fact that much of sleepiness is a result of

Table 7
Relative Cost of Diagnostic Strategies for OSA (Estimated)

Questionnaire-based likelihood assessment	1
Oximetry performed at the bedside or at home[a,b]	7
Unattended simple monitoring of cardiopulmonary channels[b]	17
Attended monitoring of sleep and cardiopulmonary variables	100

[a]Superiority over questionnaires alone not proven.
[b]Uncertainty if the patient slept and retest likely in 20–50% of unselected cases.

lifestyle rather than apneic activity, the primary care physician is in the position to advise on sleep hygiene and to allow the patient to take steps to improve his or her quality and quantity of sleep.

Deciding upon which sleep study to use for monitoring breathing and oxygenation during sleep must take into account the study accuracy and cost, as well as what is available in the local area (Table 7). In the obvious case in which the primary care provider strongly suspects OSA (the patient has excessive daytime sleepiness, loud obnoxious snoring, and hypertension), a sleep study in a place that can also start therapy will permit the most rapid institution of effective therapy. Whether this can be performed with accuracy and in a cost-effective manner in the out-patient arena such as the patient's home remains to be determined. Some health care vendors want to place sleep and breathing monitoring in the hands of people who do not have a broad range of experience with sleep disorders. It should be noted that there can be uncertain results with many studies, and some 20% of all patients found to have sleep apnea also have other sleep problems. Repeated studies are expensive and confusing to the patient. Other conditions, like restless legs syndrome (RLS), might need to be addressed before complete therapeutic success.

Sleep specialists and sleep centers that focus on the diagnosis and treatment of the broad range of sleep disorders are a resource to the primary care physician, because they combine specific medical expertise with information and education for patients. Many of these centers offer counseling or patient-oriented groups that allow the patient to understand more of his or her illness and to take better control of many basic problems—alcohol use, weight issues, or drug dependencies, as well as the potential technical problems of testing and treatment. Certainly, one of the most valuable and cost-effective steps in secondary evaluation of the sleep apnea patient is the sleep specialist (more than the sleep test). He or she is usually in the best position to decide with the patient the degree to which testing is needed prior to treatment and the exact treatment protocol. The application of nasal CPAP, for example,

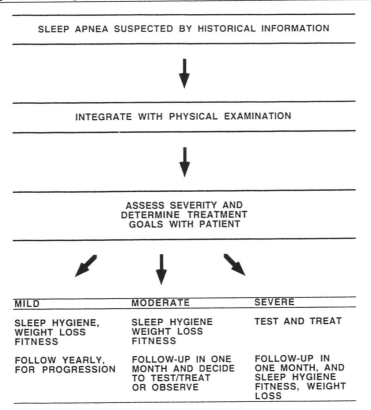

SLEEP APNEA SUSPECTED BY HISTORICAL INFORMATION

INTEGRATE WITH PHYSICAL EXAMINATION

ASSESS SEVERITY AND
DETERMINE TREATMENT
GOALS WITH PATIENT

MILD	MODERATE	SEVERE
SLEEP HYGIENE, WEIGHT LOSS FITNESS	SLEEP HYGIENE WEIGHT LOSS FITNESS	TEST AND TREAT
FOLLOW YEARLY, FOR PROGRESSION	FOLLOW-UP IN ONE MONTH AND DECIDE TO TEST/TREAT OR OBSERVE	FOLLOW-UP IN ONE MONTH, AND SLEEP HYGIENE FITNESS, WEIGHT LOSS

Fig. 3. Scheme for OSA recognition via historical information.

is done differently by different centers and physicians—some with several sleep studies per patient and some with almost none. At this point, although it is difficult to recommend the best CPAP application protocol for all patients, it is certainly best for the CPAP to be prescribed and monitored by a physician experienced with sleep and breathing problems, and most primary care physicians prefer to refer the patient who might need CPAP to a center with experience and educational resources. However, as described elsewhere in this volume, any competent physician who devotes time to education and training and who gains experience can become adept at managing many common sleep disorders.

8. MANAGEMENT CONSIDERATIONS

In the next few years, we will begin to articulate and define the relative usefulness of the various therapies in the management of all classes from this common disease. Figure 3 is an attempt to conceptualize the major management considerations by dividing patients into those who

> Although there are many treatments available for obstructive sleep apnea of various degrees of severity, nasal CPAP should be considered the "gold standard" for treatment.

are mild, moderate, or severe by whatever parameter one uses to assess the OSA. At the present time, specific treatment directed at excessive sleepiness, nocturnal angina, and cardiorespiratory failure is of highest priority. Likewise, simple snoring itself can be managed by a variety of methods including referral for surgical intervention, that do not require as intense an evaluation. However, a large number of patients fall between these two extremes, and clinical judgment and individualization of therapy is necessary. All patients will need continuing preventive care, including follow-up with regard to sleep hygiene, fitness, and reductions in cardiac risk.

9. SPECIFIC TREATMENT OPTIONS

Options available are listed in Table 8. Their various strengths and weaknesses are commented upon. As mentioned above, the exact threshold at which OSA must be treated to reduce medical risk is not certain, but treatment is desirable with any level of OSA, if the patient has problems with daytime alertness. In patients in whom the social aspect of snoring is the main target symptom, position therapy, laser-assisted uvuloplasty, nasal measures, and various snoring devices are not unreasonable to recommend, as long as one can ascertain that they pose no appreciable risk to the patient. Weight gain always worsens snoring and sleep apnea; weight loss improves snoring and OSA up to a point but is not always curative.

Nasal CPAP is continuous positive pressure applied to the nares; this treatment has become the standard treatment for OSA. It is not unreasonable to utilize CPAP for almost any level of severity of OSA. It must be stressed, that except for tracheotomy, CPAP is the most effective treatment option available and works in almost all of the patients every time, if the patient wears it. Compliance at home is not as good as it is in the laboratory, but there are still many reasons why CPAP is the treatment of choice in a majority of patients with OSA. Nasal CPAP application is an ideal way to relieve OSA, at the same time posing virtually no risk to the patient. Symptoms caused by OSA should be relieved after the patient can wear CPAP essentially all night every night for at least two weeks. Symptoms not relieved after such a trial eliminate OSA as a contributing cause. There are a variety of masks, tubing,

Table 8
Treatment Options for Moderate and Severe OSA[a]

Treatment	Problems and risks	Physiologic results	Prevention of death or disability	Patient acceptance, cost, availability
Weight loss: Medical or surgical	Selection crucial; must be able to comply, slow to achieve	10% reduction in weight can improve OSA, but results vary	Symptoms improve but outcome unproven	A lifestyle change; close follow-up
Positional therapy	Partially effective and variable	Some reduction in snoring and OSA	Unproven	Low risk, low cost intervention
Dental appliances	TMJ, gum and teeth soreness	15–55% success for one year	Unproven	Requires medical follow-up, moderate cost
CPAP	Comfort of mask, attitude adjustments by patient and spouse, noisy, cumbersome	95% success in laboratory, 60–85% long-term adherence to therapy	Yes	Available; covered by insurance but considered durable medical goods; requires education and support; must be worn nightly
Surgery on nasal septum	Risks of surgery: anesthesia and post-operative complications	Unproven	Unproven	Available, can be used as an adjunct to CPAP

UPPP	Risks of surgery, apneas become silent	Reduction of OSA in 50% of patients	Deaths not prevented (limited data)	Available; swallowing and speech affected in 2%, will require re-testing and CPAP in 50%
Mandibular advancement	Risks of surgery	Often used after UPPP failure, results vary	Unproven	Available in few centers
Medications: progesterone and serotonin-reuptake blocker	Variable effectiveness in obesity and in mild sleepiness	Results vary	Unproven	Available; costly; for use in highly selected cases
Tracheostomy	Risks of surgery; extensive postoperative care	Yes	Yes	Will require one year of adaptation by patient

[a]CPAP refers to continuous positive pressure applied to the nares. UPPP is uvulopalatopharyngoplasty, which involves reconstruction of the naso- and oropharynx.

and machine types available. All these devices blow room air into the nose to produce a positive pressure in the oropharynx, thus splinting the airway during the negative pressure of the inspiration. Functionally, CPAP acts like a tracheostomy. (*See* Chapter 10, Appendix 2, for a list of CPAP manufacturers.)

There are different algorithms to determine the best pressure setting for the device (usually in the range of 5–15 cm H_2O), and often, a sleep study in which the pressure is titrated against apneic activity is desirable. The role of the sleep study is to determine if the pressure setting is high enough to achieve adequate airway patency during inspiration, to provide a good "first time" experience to the patient, and to ascertain that no adverse reaction occurs. However, whether a laboratory study is necessary in all patients is debatable, and some specialists feel that an experienced physician and home CPAP team can supply and adjust the device adequately under direction from the patient and the bedpartner. CPAP is widely available and usually purchased from a home care company under the prescription of a physician. Common side effects include nasal congestion, rhinitis, leaking of air out the mouth, and discomfort from the mask itself. In some, the use of CPAP is objectionable, because of lifestyle or nonspecific reasons. These problems can usually be improved with common sense medical interventions, adjustment of the pressures, and attempts at better mask fit. Bilevel CPAP allows for different pressures during the inspiratory and expiratory phases of the respiratory cycle. Bilevel CPAP is often more comfortable for the patient, produces less nasal congestion and less mouth leakage, but the machines are currently larger, louder, and more expensive than CPAP machines.

Uvulopalatopharyngoplasty (UPPP) is a surgical procedure in which the soft palate is reconstructed. Its success rate for cure of OSA is probably on the order of 50%. It is probably best used in conjunction with other procedures such as hyoid suspension, and only after careful assessment of the patient's options, and attendant risk-benefit analysis. This procedure is probably the most common surgery performed for OSA in the past, but it is less commonly seen now. More extensive surgical procedures include advancement of the maxilla and mandible, a procedure with a higher degree of success but has a more limited application. Certainly, the decision to have surgery should involve a physician with broad experience in the treatment of OSA. Almost any patient considering surgery should have a trial on CPAP, and many feel that the perioperative course is safer, if the patient is on CPAP up to the time of surgery, and in the immediate postoperative period. As mentioned above, CPAP trials are also important in any patient in whom the relationship of the sleep-disordered breathing to the symptoms is in doubt—that is, one must be sure of the potential benefit to relieving apnea before proceeding with any surgical risk. In many cases of mild and moderate sleep-disordered breathing, a trial on CPAP will clarify which symptoms can be relieved and which cannot.

Dental devices that protrude or reposition the jaw have the potential to allow for a greater volume at the posterior airway space. Studies show promise for the various devices that accomplish this and are a reasonable option for mild-to-moderate OSA. Although such devices can now be purchased in pharmacies that are of the "boil and bite" type, their effect is inconsistent. Our experience is that they are poorly tolerated over time, and they can delay effective therapy. Customized models with varying mechanisms for jaw repositioning are available from selected dentists who have experience with these devices. Follow-up of patient symptoms, compliance, and a need for follow-up studies ascertained. Check the Internet or a local dental association for the Sleep Disorders Dental Society, which can often recommend a local resource.

Without question, all physicians will be seeing patients in the office who have sleep-disordered breathing and OSA. In the practice of medicine, the identification and treatment of these patients is one of the most gratifying for patient and physician alike.

CASE STUDY

The patient was a 68-year-old man with a history of coronary artery disease including a coronary artery bypass graft four years ago, hypertension, and noninsulin-dependent diabetes, who presented following the onset of substernal chest pain the morning of admission. Chest pain was substernal with radiation to the jaw and had been occurring for about one month with increasing frequency. Usually, the chest pain was present in the morning upon arising, but sometimes it occurred during the night. He was admitted for unstable angina.

Earlier in the month, he had had a coronary angiogram that showed patent saphenous vein grafts to the right coronary artery (RCA), and a patent left internal mammary artery (LIMA) to the left anterior descending artery (LAD). He had an old occlusion of the saphenous vein graft to the ramus; however, there was now an absence of collaterals to this area that has been since an angiogram two years ago. Because of the recent increase in chest pain, he was under consideration for the placement of a coronary stent; however, the increase in symptoms led to the current admission. He ruled out for myocardial infarction (MI), and supplemental oxygen, nitroglycerin, aspirin, and heparin were given. Repeat angiography showed no significant change.

A history of daytime sleepiness was obtained, as well as some insomnia and some snoring. Physical examination was unremarkable—the patient was not obese and had no obvious facial, mandibular, or oral abnormalities. An overnight oximetry in the hospital showed 153 desaturation events, as low as 75%. Polysomnography was arranged for the following night, and demonstrated about 100 apneas in the first three hours of the recording, desaturating as low as 71%. The apneas were rather impressive, lasting 40–60 seconds with prominent paradoxing of chest and abdominal motions, ending with arousal. In the second half of the study, nasal CPAP was administered, and pressures in the 6–7 cm H_2O range were markedly effective in eliminating events and in stabilizing oxyhemoglobin.

The patient was given CPAP for home use and was able to use it with great benefit. The morning chest pain was eliminated, he slept better, and he enjoyed increased daytime alertness. He was continued on an anti-anginal medical regimen. He did well for four years before being readmitted for unstable angina. Repeat cardiac catheterization showed no significant change. He continues to use his nasal CPAP all night, every night.

SUGGESTED READINGS

Chuo W, Chediak AD. Obstructive sleep apnea. Treatment improves quality of life—and may prevent death. *Postgrad Med* 1994; 95: 123–138.

Ferber R, Millman R, Coppola M, Fleetham J, Murray CF, Iber C, McCall V, Nino-Murcia G, Pressman M, Sanders M, Strohl K, Votteri B, Williams A. ASDA standards of practice: portable recording in the assessment of obstructive sleep apnea. *Sleep* 1994; 17(4): 378–392.

Leger D. The cost of sleep-related accidents: a report for the National Commission on Sleep Disorders Research. *Sleep* 1994; 17: 84–93.

National Commission on Sleep Disorders Research. *Wake Up America: A National Sleep Alert.* Volumes 1 and 2, Public Health Service, Washington, DC, 1995.

National Institutes of Health. *Sleep Apnea: Is Your Patient at Risk?* Publication No. 95-3803, Bethesda, MD, 1995.

Strohl KP, Cherniack NS, Gothe B. Physiological basis of therapy for sleep apnea. *Am Rev Respir Dis* 1986; 134: 791–802.

Strohl KP, Redline S. Recognition of obstructive sleep apnea. *Am J Resp Crit Care Med* 1996; 154: 279–289.

Tousignant P, Cosio MG, Levy RD, Groome PA. Quality adjusted life year as added by treatment of obstructive sleep apnea. *Sleep* 1994; 17: 52–60.

7

Pharmacology in Sleep Medicine

Wallace B. Mendelson and Cosmo Caruso

CONTENTS

1. INTRODUCTION

In sleep disorders, as in all of medicine, the prescription of drugs is often an integral component of treatment. This chapter focuses on two general types of sleep medications: drugs that promote sleep and drugs that promote alertness. These have been generally labeled hypnotic-sedatives and central nervous system (CNS) stimulants, respectively. There are numerous classes of agents in each category, and often, numerous specific agents in each class. A few of them are described below, separated into those generally useful in insomnia and those generally useful in states of hypersomnolence such as narcolepsy. More detailed descriptions of the clinical conditions are available elsewhere in this volume, specifically in Chapters 2 and 5.

2. MEDICATIONS FOR INSOMNIA

Insomnia, the subjective experience of inadequate quality or quantity of sleep, may have many causes. The sleep disturbance might be caused

From: *Sleep Disorders: Diagnosis and Treatment*
Edited by: J. S. Poceta and M. M. Mitler © Humana Press Inc., Totowa, NJ

by pain or other consequences of medical diseases, psychiatric disturbances such as depression, side effects of medication, circadian rhythm
disorders, or primary disorders of sleep such as central sleep apnea. In
general, the best therapeutic option for insomnia is to identify and treat
the underlying disorder. Thus, if a patient who complains of disturbed
sleep is found to have depression, the correct intervention is to admin-
ister an antidepressant; if pain from arthritis keeps a patient awake, the
best sleep aid may be an analgesic. Similarly, changing the dose or
discontinuing a medication that disturbs sleep (e.g., a beta blocker, ste-
roid, or thyroid preparation) may be the appropriate step. In many cases,
however, such causes as these cannot be found, and one must deal with
the difficulty of working with patients in whom the basic pathophysiology is poorly understood. According to the International Classification
of Sleep Disorders, this remaining group of patients can be considered
to have a "primary insomnia," usually a condition such as psychophysiological insomnia or sleep-state misperception. In the former condition,
it is thought that the patient has developed conditioned responses to
disturbed sleep (e.g., excessive worrying about not sleeping) that per-
petuate the problem. In the latter, polygraphic recordings show relatively undisturbed sleep, which is at variance with the patient's
subjective experience of sleeping very poorly or for a very short time.
The therapeutic armamentarium for dealing with these difficult types of
insomnia consists of two general approaches:

1. The administration of sedative/hypnotic medications.
2. Behaviorally oriented therapy.

This chapter will focus on the pharmacological treatment of insomnia. However, it should be noted that we do not view the two approaches
an antithetical, and there is growing evidence that a combination of both
may ultimately turn out to be particularly useful.

2.1. Neurochemical Actions of Sedative-Hypnotics

One of the challenges in psychopharmacology has been how to
explain the mechanism by which compounds from a wide variety of
chemical classes act to enhance sleep. A major step in understanding the
actions of benzodiazepines (compounds of which Valium™ is a proto-
type) came with the discovery that labeled diazepam binds to high
affinity saturable stereospecific sites in the CNS (Squires and Braestrup,
1977; Mohler and Okada, 1977). These central receptors are found in
greatest density in the synaptosomal fraction of neurons, implying that
they play a role in neurotransmission. They are thought to be pentomeric
glycoprotein structures that are comprised of three distinct but interact-

ing entities: a benzodiazepine recognition site, a GABA recognition site, and a chloride ion channel. More recent studies have revealed that the receptor complex is derived from alpha, beta, and gamma subunits, each of which have multiple isoforms. The alpha subunit determines subtype selectivity and is crucial to the binding of benzodiazepines. The beta subunit mediates the allosteric interaction with GABA, and the gamma subunit is needed for a fully functional response in terms of chloride channel activity.

The original description of the central benzodiazepine receptor complex suggested a close correlation between the affinities of various benzodiazepines for the central recognition site and their effectiveness as anxiolytics, anticonvulsants, and muscle relaxants (Squires and Braestrup, 1977). A major focus of work in our laboratory has been to examine the interaction of the central benzodiazepine receptor complex with a variety of sedative/hypnotics in sleep enhancement. In summary, these studies indicated that interaction with the benzodiazepine recognition site does indeed mediate the sleep-enhancing effects of benzodiazepines such as triazolam and flurazepam. The newer nonbenzodiazepine hypnotic zolpidem also binds at the recognition site, primarily to the Type I subtype. There are also data that indicate binding of pentobarbital to the area of the chloride ionophore of the receptor complex, and data that show that ethanol influences the behavior of the ionophore (Mendelson, 1992). For these reasons, we believe that this receptor complex may be a common site by which these diverse groups of compounds act to enhance sleep. We will examine clinical pharmacological properties of the commonly used sedative/hypnotics, and explore how to choose among them, and how they may be used most beneficially in patients with sleep disturbances.

2.2. Benzodiazepines

The benzodiazepine compounds are widely used as anticonvulsants, muscle relaxants, and sedative/hypnotics. They are named after their chemical structure, which results from a benzene ring attached to a seven-sided diazepine nucleus. Additional moieties lead to them being divided into 2-keto, 3-hydroxy, and triazolo groups. Most are completely absorbed from the gastrointestinal (GI) tract. They are very lipid soluble; among those with the most rapid onset of action are diazepam, lorazepam, alprazolam, and triazolam. They are metabolized by glucuronidation, and many have active metabolites, although the 3-hydroxy (oxazepam, lorazepam, and temazepam) and triazolo (alprazolam, triazolam) compounds do not. As seen in Tables 1 and 2, they vary greatly in elimination phase half-life, from relatively short half-lives of two to five hours

Table 1
Hypnotic/Sedatives: Benzodiazepines

Name	Trade name(s)	Elimination half-life and ~t1/2 in hours	Metabolites	Usual dosage (mg)
Alprazolam	Xanax	12–15	none	.25–.5 mg 3 ×/d (1)
Chlordiazepoxide	Librium	5–30	b,d,e,f	5–10 mg 3–4 ×/d (1)
Clonazepam	Klonopin	18–50	none	.5 mg 3 ×/d (1)
Diazepam	Valium	20–50	b,c,f	2–5 mg 2–4 ×/d (1)
Estazolam	Prosom	10–24	none	0.5–2 mg
Flurazepam	Dalmane	48–120	a,h	15–30 mg
Lorazepam	Ativan	10–20	none	1 mg 2–3 ×/d (1)
Oxazepam	Serax	3–21	none	10–15 mg 3–4 ×/d (1)
Quazepam	Doral	25–41	g,i	7.5–15 mg
Temazepam	Restoril	10–20	none	7.5–30 mg
Triazolam	Halcion	1.6–5.4	none	0.125–0.25 mg

1, Anxiolytic dose. Metabolites: [a]N-1-Hydroxyethylflurazepam (2–4); [b]Oxazepam (3–21); [c]3-Hydroxydiazepam (5–20); [d]Demoxepam (14–95); [e]Desmethylchlordiazepoxide (18); [f]Desmethyldiazepam (30–200); [g]2-Oxoquazepam (40); [h]Desalkylfluraxepam (47–100); [i]N-Desalkyl-2-oxoquazepam (70–75).

140

Table 2
Hypnotic/Sedatives: Nonbenzodiazepine Hypnotics

Drug	Name	Half-life (hours)	Dose (mg)
Pentobarbital	Nembutal	33.5	100–200
Chloral hydrate		5–9.5	500–1000
Zolpidem	Ambien	1.5–2.4	5–10 age > 65; 10–20 age < 65
Zopiclone			3.75 age > 65; 7.5 age < 65

(triazolam) to long half-lives of up to 100 hours or longer (diazepam, chlordiazepoxide, flurazepam).

One concern about the use of the long half-life compounds is that they can accumulate in the bloodstream during chronic administration, leading to daytime sedation and raising concerns about secondary consequences such as falls in the elderly or automobile accidents. Basic pharmacological principles remind us that the steady-state plasma level of a compound is not reached until about five half-lives of administration. Thus, for a drug with a half-life of 72 hours, plasma levels from daily dosing will continue to rise for about two weeks. The shorter-acting agents are relatively free from this problem, which was a major reason for their rapid acceptance by the medical community when they were introduced in the early 1980s. Although there have been allegations from some investigators that the very short-acting triazolam may cause an increased rate of other types of daytime difficulties, including anxiety or amnesiac states, our interpretation of the literature is that with recommended doses, these effects are not more likely than with other benzodiazepine hypnotics. A recent review of experience during a three-year period in a 1000-bed teaching hospital suggests that for benzodiazepines as a whole, reported adverse reactions occurred with benzodiazepines at rates ranging from .05% (lorazepam) to none (chlorazepate) per dose administered, with a mean of .01% of doses administered (Mendelson, 1997A). The rate for triazolam was .02%. Of particular concern in the use of sedative/hypnotics is that they may lead to patient falls. A recent study found that hospitalized patients who sustained a fall were 2.7 times more likely to have received a psychotropic medication (Mendelson, 1997B). In this study, benzodiazepines that were statistically associated with falls included temazepam, alprazolam, diazepam, and lorazepam.

CNS depressants of almost any type can have an additive effect with the benzodiazepines, thus, should be administered with extreme caution. Consequently, anticonvulsants and alcohol may greatly increase sedation from these compounds. In fact, there are a number of drug–drug interactions involving the benzodiazepines. For example, when disulfiram is used in combination with benzodiazepines, a reduction in dosage may be required. Cimetidine also may reduce the plasma clearance of benzodiazepines through inhibition of hepatic microsomal enzymes, leading to increased duration of action of the sedative. One study revealed a decrease in clearance of triazolam when administered with erythromycin. The use of antacids with chlordiazepoxide or diazepam may decrease the rate of absorption. Dioxin levels may need to be monitored when given in combination with certain benzodiazepines, such as diazepam or alprazolam.

2.2.1. TRIAZOLAM

Triazolam is rapidly absorbed, does not have an active metabolite and has an elimination half-life of 1.6–5.4 hours. Usually, elimination is more rapid in younger subjects and is more prolonged in older subjects. Triazolam has potent hypnotic properties that are evident on the first night of administration, and many (though not all) studies have shown no evidence of tolerance to polygraphic measures of sleep enhancement after one month of administration (Mendelson, 1995). Because of its short elimination half-life, it does not produce daytime residual sedation. Although one laboratory has reported increases in daytime anxiety during its use, a number of subsequent studies have found no evidence to suggest this phenomenon. Again, as a consequence of its short half-life, however, there may be transient sleep disturbance when high doses are discontinued. This phenomenon is dose-related and can be avoided by using lower doses and by tapering the dose for two or three nights before stopping. Thus, a patient taking .25 mg can be placed successfully on .125 mg briefly to minimize this problem. To illustrate the importance of determining the underlying cause of a patient's sleep complaint, triazolam 0.25 mg has been studied in patients with severe obstructive sleep apnea; it produced modest increases in event duration and decreases in arterial oxygen desaturation (Berry et al., 1995).

2.2.2. ESTAZOLAM

One of the intermediate-acting agents, estazolam is readily absorbed, with peak plasma concentrations within two hours, and it has an elimination half-life of 10–24 hours. One study of elderly subjects has suggested that plasma concentrations are similar to those of younger patients, with a mean half-life of 18.4 hours. Even though estazolam does not have a long-acting active metabolite, because of its half-life, there will be accumulation with continued use, and some daytime somnolence may be observed. An initial dose of 0.5 mg may be used in the elderly or debilitated and increased with caution.

2.2.3. TEMAZEPAM

Temazepam is readily absorbed, and after a 30 mg dose, the peak plasma levels occur 1.2–1.6 hours after ingestion. Some authors have suggested that because of the slow time-to-peak concentration, temazepam may be better used for sleep-maintenance insomnia. An initial dose of 7.5 mg may be sufficient for patients with transient or mild insomnia. The dose may be given approximately 30 minutes before retiring, and the usual precautions regarding benzodiazepine effects should be given. In Great Britain, there have been reports of cases of intra-arterial injection of an "abuse-resistant" preparation of temazepam; apparently abusers remove the gelatin shell, boil the gel center, and inject the suspension. In some cases, this has resulted in severe pain and medical complications requiring amputation. In fact, all the benzodiazepines are capable of being used incorrectly, abused in order to achieve an altered mental state, especially in susceptible populations.

2.2.4. FLURAZEPAM

This compound, the oldest benzodiazepine recommended as a hypnotic, is long-acting, producing an active metabolite with a half-life of 40–100 hours or longer. There may be impaired clearance in the elderly and in patients with hepatic disorders. As previously mentioned, because of its long half-life, there may be significant accumulation over time, with resulting daytime sedation. Sometimes, this can be used to advantage, such as allowing for some antianxiety effect during the day, or in achieving a slow "self-taper" when the agent is discontinued. The usual dose is 15–30 mg.

2.2.5. QUAZEPAM

Quazepam is one of the long-acting benzodiazepine agents, with an active metabolite that may predispose to residual daytime sedation. The initial dose in the elderly and debilitated should be 7.5 mg. A double-blind study comparing quazepam and triazolam in 45 patients with generalized anxiety disorder and insomnia showed that anxiety improved with both drugs and continued improved after two weeks (Saletu et al., 1994). Awakenings improved in both groups; however, somatic complaints did not improve with triazolam. Psychometric testing in the morning showed improved attention with both medications.

2.3. Nonbenzodiazepine Hypnotics

2.3.1. CHLORAL HYDRATE

Chloral hydrate is rapidly absorbed, and doses of 500 mg to 1 g typically induce sleep in 30–60 minutes. The active metabolite is trichloroethanol. Rapid eye movement (REM) rebound has been reported to be minimal during withdrawal of this agent. Chloral hydrate can be irritating to the GI tract, and rare adverse reactions such as nausea, vomiting, diarrhea, unpleasant taste, drowsiness, ataxia, and leukopenia may be seen. It is contraindicated in patients with hepatic or renal impairment. The drug crosses the placenta and may cause sedation in breast-feeding infants. Its toxicity in acute overdose is similar to that of barbiturates.

2.3.2. BARBITURATES

Although the medium-duration barbiturates such as pentobarbital and secobarbital are potent hypnotics, their toxicity compared to newer agents limits their utility for insomnia to rare selected patients. They have a small therapeutic range, significant addiction potential, respiratory suppressant properties, and are lethal in overdose. Barbiturates cause reduced REM and slow wave sleep, although the clinical significance of these sleep-stage alterations is uncertain. REM rebound occurs with withdrawal of the drug, and the patient may experience disturbed sleep and/or vivid dreaming. These compounds are slowly metabolized by hepatic microsomal enzymes and may increase the rate of breakdown of concomitantly administered drugs that undergo hepatic metabolism. Barbiturates are contraindicated in pregnancy and lactation. The drug interactions include CNS depressants, corticosteroids, anticoagulants, and oral contraceptives.

2.3.3. ZOPICLONE

Zopiclone, a cyclopyrrolone, is available for clinical use in Europe and in Canada but not in the U.S. Although a nonbenzodiazepine, its therapeutic actions are thought to derive from interacting with the benzodiazepine-GABA receptor complex. Peak plasma concentrations are achieved within two hours. Bioavailability is approximately 80%, but it is increased in the elderly. There is extensive hepatic metabolism; plasma zopiclone clearance is not altered by hemodialysis. The elimination half-life is 3.5–6.5 hours in young volunteers, compared to eight hours in older subjects. There are varying effects on duration of REM sleep. Although some studies revealed only mild respiratory depression, zopiclone has been shown to increase the apnea index in patients with an apnea index greater than 20 per hour.

2.3.4. ZOLPIDEM

Zolpidem is an imidazopyridine derivative. It has been shown to act at the Type I subtype of the GABA-benzodiazepine receptor–chloride ionophore complex. This may be the reason that zolpidem has a greater sleep-inducing effect relative to any muscle relaxation, anticonvulsant, or anxiolytic effect. It has a rapid onset of action of approximately 15–30 minutes. The plasma elimination phase half-life is approximately 2.4 hours, making it a short-acting hypnotic. Sleep architecture studies have shown minimal changes in stage 2, with no change or an increase in slow wave sleep. There are minimal effects on REM sleep. Withdrawal sleep disturbance appears to be minimal (Monti et al., 1994). Like the benzodiazepines, it may have mild respiratory depressant qualities in patients with preexisting sleep apnea (Cirignotta et al., 1988). The most common side effects that have resulted in discontinuation involve the GI and nervous systems. The most frequent GI side effects are diarrhea, nausea, and dyspepsia; drowsiness and dizziness have been the most frequent CNS difficulties. Myalgia, arthralgia, palpitation, rash, sinusitis, and pharyngitis have also been reported.

Residual daytime effects from zolpidem have been minimal. A reduced dose should be given to patients with liver disease, and dosage adjustment in renal disease may be necessary. Older patients may have an increase in the peak plasma concentration and half-life, and an initial reduction in dose is appropriate. The typical adult dose of zolpidem tartrate is 10 mg—5 mg for older patients.

2.3.5. ANTIHISTAMINES

The active ingredients in most over-the-counter (OTC) sleep aids are the sedating antihistamines, diphenhydramine hydrochloride or doxylamine succinate. They probably should not be recommended to any patient with an insomnia problem great enough to be seeking physician advice. Although these agents are well documented for producing daytime sleepiness as measured by the Multiple Sleep Latency Test, there are less data on efficacy as nighttime hypnotics than might be desired. Their anticholinergic properties can be problematic, and they have been shown to induce decrements in dexterity, memory, and concentration. Some of the side effects with certain OTC sleep aids include blurred vision, constipation, morning sedation, tinnitus, dizziness, and palpitations.

2.3.1. ANTIDEPRESSANTS

The tricyclic antidepressants are a heterogeneous group of compounds comprised of tertiary and secondary amines. They are marketed as antidepressants but are sometimes used "off-label" to help sleep.

They are only moderately well absorbed, and there is significant first-pass metabolism. The tertiary compounds are demethylated to secondary amines; the tricyclic nucleus undergoes hepatic oxidation and is excreted as a glucuronic acid conjugate. The tricyclics are generally very lipid soluble. Most have half-lives of 10–70 hours, though this can be longer for nortriptyline and protriptyline. Their actions include reduction of reuptake of norepinephrine and serotonin (in various proportions depending on the specific agent), as well as antihistaminic and anticholinergic effects. After chronic administration, there is a reduction in the number of beta-adrenergic and serotonin Type 2 receptors, which is thought to occur temporally with the onset of antidepressant therapeutic effects. Among the most frequent adverse experiences are anticholinergic effects such as dry mouth, increased heart rate, and urinary hesitancy. Amitriptyline is among the most anticholinergic; nortriptyline and desipramine are among the least. There is significant cardiac toxicity in acute overdose. In addition, they probably should not be used intermittently or "as needed," and nightly administration is usual.

The tricyclics have two types of roles in the treatment of insomnia:

1. If examination of the patient suggests that the sleep disturbance is secondary to major depressive disorder, the appropriate treatment is an antidepressant, including the tricyclics;
2. They are useful as drugs of second choice in patients with primary insomnia who have not responded to traditional sedative/hypnotics. The major concerns about their use are their long half-lives, significant toxicity in overdose, and their anticholinergic side effects. When administered for insomnia, a sedating tricyclic such as amitriptyline is typically given in low doses such as 10 to 50 mg.

The selective serotonin reuptake inhibitors (SSRIs) do not have potent sedative effects, but they are an indispensable component in treating depression. Paroxetine is probably the most sedating of the group, but it can only be considered an adjunct in treating a primary insomnia. Fluoxetine commonly produces a sleep complaint and sometimes needs to be combined with a sedating agent.

Trazodone, a triazolopyridine derivative marketed as an antidepressant, is sometimes used to aid sleep as an off-label indication. In one trial, trazodone significantly reduced the frequency of sleep arousals and REM sleep time and increased slow wave sleep. One case report has described the utility of trazodone for treating sleep terror disorder and insomnia (Balon, 1994). Monoamine oxidase inhibitors (MAOIs) have been known to cause delay in sleep onset, which has caused some patients to discontinue their use. Trazodone has been used concomitantly in this situation in low doses (50 to 100 mg) to improve medication-induced insomnia. A study of six middle-aged subjects with chronic insomnia associated with dysthymia reported an increase of slow wave sleep with reduction in stage 2 sleep throughout the treatment period with trazodone CR. The changes in sleep architecture were associated with improvement in scores on visual analog scales of sleep quality and the Hamilton rating scale for depression.

3. EFFECTS OF MEDICATIONS ON SLEEP

Having reviewed a variety of agents that can be used to aid sleep, we will now consider the converse issue: that many medications used to treat illnesses may result in sleep disturbance. When confronted with a patient with chronic insomnia, one of the first steps should be to consider whether the problem could result from a medication, and if so, to alter the dose or discontinue use if possible. A detailed analysis of each agent is beyond the scope of this text; often, there is incomplete knowledge of the exact mechanisms involved.

Beta adrenoreceptor antagonists have been reported to cause hallucinations, dreaming, disturbed sleep, tiredness, and drowsiness. A differentiation should be made between these CNS effects and actions on cardiovascular function as a cause of the patient's fatigue. The lipophilic compounds such as propranolol seem to be implicated more often in sleep complaints. Beta-2 agonists, commonly used to treat asthma, have clinical effectiveness for approximately for three to four hours; thus, patients sometimes awaken with symptoms as a result of their disorder in the latter part of the night. Theophylline preparations vary with regard to their duration of action, and timing of dose should be addressed in patients with asthma and COPD. Clearly, theophylline is a stimulant. The histamine-2 antagonist cimetidine has been reported to increase slow wave sleep; drowsiness has been described in patients with renal and liver problems.

Clonidine, an alpha-2 adrenoreceptor agonist, has been shown to increase stage 2 and the total sleep time. Drowsiness, vivid dreams, nightmares, and insomnia have been reported. The drowsiness may ameliorate with time and/or reduction in dose; however, this may continue and require discontinuation of the drug. The timing of diuretic administration in relation to sleep time should be considered in assessing patients who awaken from sleep with the urge to urinate. Hypolipidemic agents such as lovastatin and simvastatin have been associated with insomnia.

CNS stimulants such as amphetamines, pemoline, and methylphenidate have been reported to disrupt sleep. Methylphenidate, in contrast to pemoline, seems to increase wakefulness at night and reduce REM sleep. The timing of dosing of these agents is very important. Ideally, when given to patients with narcolepsy, for instance, it is best to give the last dose no later than noon, if possible. Other drugs that can disturb sleep include calcium channel blockers, thyroid preparations, anticonvulsants, and cancer chemotherapeutic agents.

Opioids, such as morphine, induce a state of relaxed wakefulness with relatively less increase in physiologic sleep than is often thought. They potently decrease REM sleep. There may be increased arousals and stage 1 sleep with some of these agents.

The effects of caffeine on sleep may be caused by antagonistic effects on adenosine receptors. Caffeine causes increased wakefulness and reduction in total sleep time, slow wave sleep, and REM sleep. These effects may last for greater than eight hours. All patients evaluated for a sleep problem should have their daily consumption of caffeinated beverages assessed. Little is known about the effects that nicotine has on sleep. It has been suggested that at high concentrations, it may cause arousal and at low blood levels, sedation. Further study is warranted, but a history of the patient's use and time of use of nicotine should be investigated. Nicotine withdrawal syndrome often includes insomnia and fatigue.

Alcohol is very commonly used as a form of self-medication to aid sleep. In general, although it may induce sleep, it is metabolized so rapidly that sleep in the last third of the night becomes disturbed by multiple awakenings. In chronic use, there may be decreased slow wave sleep, increased REM, and sleep disruption. During acute withdrawal, frequent arousals and awakenings are noted. When alcohol-dependent patients become "dry," sleep difficulties can continue for years. Patients with chronic obstructive pulmonary disease (COPD) may have more nocturnal hypoxemia and ventricular arrhythmias after alcohol ingestion; similarly, sleep apnea may be exacerbated.

4. MEDICATIONS FOR EXCESSIVE SLEEPINESS

Psychostimulants have been used for years in tonics and other preparations to treat fatigue, sleepiness, and other ailments. Coffee might be the most common stimulant now generally used. Ephedrine was an early treatment of narcolepsy, followed by the amphetamines. After 1956, methylphenidate came into broad use, as suggested by Yoss and Daly. Since the mid 1970s, the use of stimulants was modified by the introduction of REM suppressing antidepressants, newer medications, and the concomitant application of psychological and sleep hygiene advice.

Table 3
Psychomotor Stimulant Drugs

Direct sympathomimetics

Isoproterenol	Phenylephrine
Epinephrine	Apomorphine
Norepinephrine	Ephedrine

Indirect sympathomimetics

Amphetamine	Phenylpropanolamine
Cocaine	Pemoline
Mazindol	Phenmetrazine
Methamphetamine	Pipradol
Methylphenidate	Tyramine

Others

Caffeine	Scopolamine
Nicotine	Atropine
Theophylline	Strychnine
Aminophylline	Pentylenetetrazol
Modafinil	

Abuse of these agents over the last few decades has also altered prescribing and treatment approaches, but stimulants remain the cornerstone of treatment in the United States. Much of the following discussion is adapted directly from a comprehensive review of this topic by Mitler, Aldrich, Koob, and Zarcone (1994).

4.1. Pharmacology of Stimulants

Psychomotor stimulants produce behavioral activation usually accompanied by increases in arousal, motor activity, and alertness. There are three major classes of psychomotor stimulants:

1. Direct-acting sympathomimetics, such as phenylephrine.
2. Indirect-acting sympathomimetics, such as amphetamine and amphetamine-like compounds.
3. Stimulants that are not sympathomimetics and have different mechanisms of action (*see* Table 3).

Because of their numerous side effects on the peripheral nervous system, direct sympathomimetics are not used in clinical practice. Most compounds available for clinical use act indirectly on dopaminergic and, to a lesser extent, on adrenergic systems. We shall describe aspects of indirectly acting sympathomimetic drugs only.

Most indirect sympathomimetic compounds share a common molecular structure: a benzene ring with an ethylamine side chain. Amphetamine differs from the parent compound, beta-phenethylamine, by the addition of a methyl group, and methamphetamine has two additional methyl groups. Methylphenidate and cocaine are structurally similar. Amphetamines were originally synthesized for use as inhalants for the treatment of asthma, and they have been also used by the military as antifatigue medications. They are currently available for medical use as adjuncts for short-term weight control, attentional deficit hyperactivity disorder, and narcolepsy.

Indirect sympathomimetics act primarily by increasing the amount of monoamines available within the synaptic cleft of monoamine synapses in the central nervous system and by blocking reuptake and enhancing release of norepinephrine, dopamine, and serotonin. Amphetamines are also weak inhibitors of monoamine oxidase. The primary action responsible for the psychomotor stimulant effects of indirect sympathomimetics appears to be on the dopamine systems in the CNS. The midbrain dopamine systems include two major pathways that project to the forebrain and appear to be responsible for different aspects of psychomotor stimulant actions. The mesocorticolimbic dopamine system projects to the ventral forebrain, including the nucleus accumbens, olfactory tubercle, septum, and frontal cortex, and the nigrostriatal dopamine system arises primarily in the substantia nigra and projects to the corpus striatum.

4.2. Pharmacokinetics

Oral and intravenous doses of amphetamines increase blood pressure and heart rate, although higher doses may induce a reflex slowing of heart rate. Amphetamines produce bronchial and pupillary dilation as well as decreases in glandular secretions. These effects are mediated by the sympathetic nervous system.

Amphetamine and related drugs are powerful stimulants of the CNS. This effects are characterized by increased wakefulness, alertness, decreased sense of fatigue, elevations of mood and euphoria, increased motor activity and talkativeness, and increased performance in some tasks and athletic situations. The CNS effects of low doses of methamphetamine are more pronounced than the autonomic effects, presumably because of increased lipophilicity, allowing it to readily cross the blood–brain barrier.

The intensity of stimulant effects of cocaine and amphetamines depends on the route of administration. Intranasal or oral administration of 2.5–15 mg d-amphetamine produces feelings of alertness, energetic vitality, confident assertiveness, and a decrease in appetite and fatigue. Intranasal absorption is faster and has more intense effects, and the stimulant effects of amphetamines last up to 4 - 6 hours. Ten milligrams or more of d-amphetamine taken intravenously or inhaled produces intense, usually pleasurable, sensations characterized as a "rush" that probably acts as a motivation for the abuse of these drugs.

Amphetamine is deaminated in the liver, oxidized to benzoic acid, and then excreted as glucoroxide or glycine conjugates. With normal pH urine, approximately 30% is excreted unchanged. Amphetamine has a half-life of approximately 12 hours, but since it has a pKa of 9.9, that half-life can be extended with an alkaline urine to over 16 hours and shortened to eight hours with acid urine. Methamphetamine reaches a peak blood concentration approximately one hour after ingestion, one hour faster than oral dextroamphetamine. Methamphetamine is the most rapidly absorbed form of amphetamine, presumably because of its lipophilicity, and has a pKa and renal excretion similar to the parent compound. Methylphenidate has a metabolic half-life of approximately two to four hours and is de-esterized to the inactive ritalinic acid and excreted in the urine. This inactivation accounts for over 80% of the removal of methylphenidate.

4.3. Clinical Application of Stimulants

Amphetamines in doses that produce stimulant effects also can enhance performance in simple (but not complex) motor and cognitive tasks, including reaction time, attention, and performance. Other reported effects include: slight enhancement of athletic performance; improved coordination, strength and endurance; increased mental and physical activation, and mood changes of boldness, elation, and friendliness. The most dramatic effects of amphetamines have been observed in situations of fatigue and boredom. Amphetamines and related compounds decrease appetite, but tolerance to this particular effect develops rapidly.

Amphetamines and methylphenidate decrease sleepiness, increase the latency to falling asleep, increase latency to the onset of REM sleep, and reduce the proportion of REM sleep. Nocturnal sleep disturbance is common, as well.

Among clinicians, there is the impression that stimulants vary in the degree to which they control sleepiness. However, it is difficult to measure objectively the relative efficacy of stimulants. Among the most important problems hampering the objective ranking of stimulants are:

1. Investigators have used different outcome measures (e.g., clinical assessment, MSLT, maintenance of wakefulness test [MWT], or other).

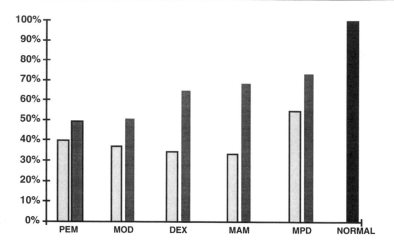

Fig. 1. Relative efficacy of stimulant drugs commonly used to treat narcolepsy. The lightest shading denotes baseline sleep latencies on either MSLT or MWT expressed in terms of percent of normal levels (13.4 minutes for the MSLT and 18.9 min for the MWT) and the darker shading denotes values observed at the highest dose of each drug evaluated. See text for methods. Abbreviations: PEM, pemoline; MOD, modafinil; DEX, dextroamphetamine; MAM, methamphetamine; MPD, methylphenidate (from Mitler and Hajdukovic, 1991).

2. Subject samples vary widely in the baseline level of sleepiness.
3. Some investigators have studied multiple doses, thereby providing a basis for estimating the dose-response curve where others have not.
4. There is little correlation between oral dose and blood level of methylphenidate and possibly of other stimulants.

In order to compare in some way the relative effects of stimulants, Mitler used a normalization technique (Mitler and Hajdukovic, 1991). This technique permitted some degree of quantitative comparison among previously published treatment efficacy studies that employed daytime polysomnographic testing (MSLT or MWT) of daytime sleepiness. The following treatment and testing conditions were compared: pemoline, 112.5 mg using the MWT; modafinil, 300 mg using the MWT; dexedrine, 60 mg using the MWT; methylphenidate, 60 mg using the MWT; and methamphetamine, 40–60 mg using the MSLT. Results are summarized in Fig. 1. The lighter bars represent mean sleep latency observed during baseline conditions and the darker bars represent mean sleep latency observed during treatment. A shorter sleep latency is indicative of more sleepiness.

Table 4
Published Recommendations
of Stimulant Dosages for Treatment of Narcolepsy

Medication	Daily dose range
Ritalin®/methylphenidate	Up to 80 mg Occasional use of up to 100–300 mg Up to 40–60 mg in children
Dextroamphetamine	Up to 60 mg
Desoxyn®/methamphetamine	5–100 mg
Cylert®/pemoline	100 mg
Mazindol	2–8 mg
Levo-amphetamine (not available in US)	20–60 mg

Although baseline measurements varied, each drug produced a clinically significant change above baseline toward normal levels. Dexedrine, methamphetamine, and methylphenidate brought measurements above 60% of normal levels; the largest change from baseline occurred with methamphetamine. However, more comparative studies with more and higher dose levels and larger numbers of subjects are needed. Ultimately, clinicians treat a patient based on his or her particular therapeutic needs and abilities to tolerate side effects. The majority of patients with narcolepsy can be adequately controlled by the use of one of these medications at a reasonable dosage. Table 4 gives published doses of medications often used in narcolepsy.

4.4. Side Effects of Stimulants

Stimulants commonly produce side effects when used in the treatment of narcolepsy or other conditions. The reported frequency of side effects of stimulants in clinical practice and in clinical trials varies greatly, depending on the method of determining a side effect and the definition of a side effect. Common side effects include headaches, irritability, nervousness or tremulousness, anorexia, insomnia, GI complaints, dyskinesias, and palpitations. In a study of 100 patients, 10% discontinued stimulants because of failure to respond, tolerance, or side effects (Parkes et al., 1975). However, in 20 narcoleptics, a trial of lower doses of dextroamphetamine—10–30 mg/d—caused no increase in side effects compared to baseline (Shindler et al., 1985). Disturbed nocturnal sleep has been reported with dexedrine, methamphetamine, and methylphenidate, especially at higher doses. Some studies have reported that the incidence of tolerance and side effects is less in narcoleptics than in others taking methylphenidate or methamphetamine, but the basis for this belief is not clear. There is little evidence that stimulants cause a clinically significant increase in blood pressure at commonly used doses in normotensive individuals, but certainly blood pressure must be followed carefully, especially in older or hypertensive patients. Side effects may be less frequent with modafinil than with amphetamines, whereas side effects with selegiline 20–30 mg/d are comparable to dextroamphetamine in similar doses. Pemoline has been reported to cause liver dysfunction.

4.5. Use of Stimulants in Children

Most of the available data on the effects of stimulants in children concern their use for attention deficit/hyperactivity disorder rather than for narcolepsy. The potential side effect of greatest concern is growth retardation (Croche et al., 1979). However, most studies have found little or no evidence of long-term effects on growth, and some have found greater than expected increases (Gross, 1976). Any effects of methylphenidate on growth in prepubertal children appear not to extend into adolescence, and, in one study, adult height of treated children was no different than height of controls or national norms. Other side effects of stimulants in the treatment of children with attention deficit/hyperactivity disorder include anorexia, insomnia, and weight loss; however, these are usually transient and diminish with continued treatment.

It appears that the incidence and severity of side effects and the overall safety of stimulants are similar in children with narcolepsy and children with attention deficit/hyperactivity disorder at comparable dosing levels. Some authorities recommend the following initial doses of stimulants for attention deficit/hyperactivity disorder: methylphenidate, 0.3 mg/kg; dextroamphetamine, 0.15 mg/kg; and pemoline, 37.5 mg, with careful titration to achieve optimal effects. The safety in narcoleptic children of higher doses than those currently recommended for attention deficit/hyperactivity disorder (e.g., methylphenidate 60 mg/d) is unknown.

4.6. Complications of Stimulants

Psychosis and hallucinations are rare in narcoleptics treated with stimulants. There have been only isolated examples of cases of amphetamine psychosis, hallucinations, and addiction. Some investigators suggest that the incidence of side effects is less with methylphenidate than with dextroamphetamine or methamphetamine.

The likelihood of psychosis or hallucinations induced by stimulants is increased in patients with coexisting psychiatric conditions. In patients with narcolepsy who develop psychosis in association with stimulant use, there is often evidence of coexisting or preexisting psychiatric illness. The relation of these complications to dose is uncertain, although many clinicians believe—and it is logical to assume—that the risk of psychiatric complications is greater at higher doses. Some have observed that hallucinatory paranoid states caused by stimulants will be less likely to occur when the patient follows a program of regular sleep habits, an afternoon nap, and a maximum dose of methylphenidate 80 mg/d or pemoline 100 mg/d.

Cardiac and vascular complications have been reported rarely in narcoleptics. There are reports of the occurrence of strokes, cardiomyopathy, and ischemic colitis, but it is not clear that these have occurred as a direct result of the medications. These complications must be assessed in light of the many narcoleptics who have taken stimulants on a regular basis for decades, often into the seventh or eighth decade of life, without developing cardiovascular disturbances. Although some clinicians consider hypertension to be a contraindication for stimulant therapy, it is often necessary to employ stimulants in narcoleptics with hypertension.

Amphetamine abuse can produce a variety of effects. Major symptoms reported of amphetamine toxicity are agitation, hallucinations, suicidal behavior, and chest pain. Seizures, intracranial hypertension, ischemic strokes, fatal and nonfatal intracranial hemorrhages, and narrowing and dilation of intracranial arteries have occurred after intravenous, intranasal, or oral abuse of amphetamine or methamphetamine. There is a strong clinical association of amphetamine drug abuse with stroke. Complications of intravenous use of amphetamines include myocardial infarction and acute left ventricular failure, mononeuropathy multiplex with angitis, acute renal failure, and drug-induced elevation of serum thyroxine. These complications are probably more common after intravenous use of large quantities of stimulants.

Although tolerance develops to many of the effects of amphetamines, the frequency and importance of tolerance to the alerting effects of stimulants in the treatment of sleepiness is controversial. Tolerance to the alerting effects of stimulants in narcoleptics appears to occur with variable frequency, in the 10–30% range. Some have found no tolerance in selected series of patients. Other investigators note that tolerance to stimulants is more likely to occur with high doses. Guilleminault (Guilleminault et al., 1974) described six patients who had increased their intake of dextroamphetamine to more than 100 mg/d because of an increase in sleep attacks and cataplexy but "in all cases, the increased amphetamine intake did not help them in any way." With lower doses, none worsened and three improved.

Although possible, there is little evidence for the view that the incidence of tolerance and side effects is less in narcoleptics than in other persons taking comparable doses. It is possible that tolerance reported by some patients is not true tolerance; rather, an effect of the narcoleptic's inadequate nocturnal sleep. Nor is it clear if the tolerance of some agents (methylphenidate) is less likely than other agents (dextroamphetamine).

5. SUMMARY: PRESCRIBING MEDICATIONS FOR PATIENTS WITH SLEEP DISORDERS

Our options for the pharmacologic treatment of many diseases are expanding. Never before have we had so many relatively safe and effective medications for so many disorders, including sleep disorders. Although there is still no "perfect sleeping pill," and no pill to completely remove sleepiness or our need for sleep, some help is available for virtually every patient with insomnia or excessive daytime sleepiness.

The following are guidelines for managing a patient with sleep disturbance who presents in a primary care setting. Medications are prescribed in the context of an understanding of the problem. Fundamentally, a series of questions need to be asked, whether the complaint is excessive sleepiness or insomnia; we focus here on insomnia. The clinical decision-making involved in the prescription of stimulants is covered in Chapter 5.

5.1. Gathering Information

What is the duration of the problem? If the patient's sleep disturbance is of only a few days' duration and seems tied to a specific emotionally upsetting event, the best intervention is reassurance, possibly coupled with a few days' supply of a hypnotic. If sleep disturbance has persisted for weeks or months and does not seem to be a reaction to a specific trauma, one would proceed with the following steps.

Could the sleep disturbance be explained by a medication the patient is taking for some other condition? If so, the response is to alter the dose or, if possible, to change to a different medication. Is there excessive use of caffeine or nicotine? If so, reduction in their consumption should be part of the regimen.

If the patient cannot sleep because of pain, the appropriate treatment might be an analgesic, not a hypnotic. If a patient cannot sleep because of orthopnea, adjustment of the cardiovascular or diuretic regimen would be in order.

Is there a major psychiatric illness present? Probably of greatest concern is depression, which often presents initially as a "somatic" complaint, such as change in appetite or weight, decreased energy or libido, or insomnia. If the patient is depressed, the appropriate treatment would be therapeutic doses of antidepressant medications such as the tricyclics. The sleep-promoting qualities of many of them, such as amitriptyline, may give the patient relief from insomnia within a night or two, even before the true antidepressant qualities are manifest (often two or three weeks later).

Is there a primary disorder of sleep? At some point in the workup, a decision will need to be made as to whether the patient should be referred to a sleep-disorders specialist for a workup of primary sleep disorders. However, the urgency of doing so hinges on the level of suspicion that such disorders are present. A series of screening questions will help with that determination; the specific questions are dependent on the illness and can be derived from the various chapters in this book. As an example, when considering periodic leg movement disorder, one would ask whether the patient's bed partner has complained of kicking movements during sleep, and whether the bedcovers are messy or neat in the morning. For obstructive sleep apnea, which is more likely to cause sleepiness but can present as a sleep disturbance complaint, one would ask about weight gain in the last few years, a history of snoring and hypertension, and whether a bed partner has witnessed possible apneic episodes.

5.2. Making A Plan

If the previous information has not yielded a plan of action (e.g., treating depression, changing dose of a medication), and if the suspicion of a primary sleep disorder is low, one would consider the use of sedative/hypnotic medication, alone or in combination with behavioral therapy. In either event, it is useful for the patient to keep a sleep diary, which documents the baseline condition as a measure of later progress. The choice of medication depends on a variety of factors; in an inpatient setting, for instance, the greater toxicity during overdose of antidepressants or the older agents, such as chloral hydrate, is not a consideration. In an outpatient setting, such potential toxicity is a very real issue, and it is better to use benzodiazepines or the newer nonbenzodiazepine agents such as zolpidem. When choosing among the benzodiazepines, the major factor in selection focuses on duration of effective action, which is reflected in the elimination half-life. If daytime sedation, in addition to improved sleep, is desired, the long-acting agents would be preferable. However, this is usually not the case, and in most circumstances, a shorter-acting benzodiazepine or zolpidem, which have fewer daytime residual effects, is more desirable. The authors' impression of the antihistamines is that although they are well documented to induce daytime sleepiness, their potency as hypnotics is slight; thus, their utility in treating chronic insomnia is limited.

If benzodiazepines or zolpidem are not effective, the tricyclic antidepressants or trazodone can be employed as drugs of second choice. Limitations of the tricyclics, as mentioned earlier, are their anticholinergic side effects, and the danger of toxicity in overdose. When giving trazodone, male patients should be cautioned about the unlikely but possible appearance of priapism.

The decision as to whether to employ behavioral therapy alone or in conjunction with pharmacotherapy is a difficult one for which there are not clear guidelines. The limited data available suggest that behavioral methods take longer to work initially but may have more lasting benefits. There is also some preliminary suggestion that the two approaches may be successfully combined. In the authors' clinic, for instance, patients are often given a prescription for a short-acting hypnotic in quantities of two or three doses per week to be used when the patient is undergoing behavioral therapy. Based on clinical experience, this seems a useful strategy, but long-term studies will be needed to confirm the efficacy of this approach.

Another major concern is whether hypnotic treatment will lose its effectiveness. The traditional teaching has been that tolerance develops for hypnotics after two or three weeks of administration. This is no longer so clear, with a number of studies indicating that effectiveness for triazolam continues throughout one-month trials and with studies of up to six months with zolpidem. Many sleep clinicians are reconsidering the issue of whether tolerance inevitably develops so quickly. In the absence of a definitive answer, the best strategy remains to use the lowest dose for the shortest possible time. Rebound insomnia is least likely to occur if the agent is long-lasting, and if the dosage of a short-acting agent is tapered before discontinuation.

REFERENCES

Balon R. Sleep terror disorder and insomnia treated with trazodone: a case report. *Ann Clin Psychia* 1994; 6: 161–163.

Berry RB, Kouchi K, Bower J, Prosise G, Light RW. Triazolam in patients with obstructive sleep apnea. *AJRCCM* 1995; 151: 450–454.

Cirignotta F, Mondini S, Zucconi M, Gerardi R, Farolfi A, Lugaresi E. Zolpidem-polysomnographic study of the effect of a new hypnotic drug in sleep apnea syndrome. *Pharm Biochem Behav* 1988; 29: 807–809.

Croche AF, Lipman RS, Overall JE, Hung W. The effects of stimulant medication on the growth of hyperkinetic children. *Pediatrics* 1979; 63: 847–850.

Daly DD, Yoss RE. The treatment of narcolepsy with methyl phenylpiperidylacetate: a preliminary report. *Proc Mayo Clin* 1956; 31: 620–625.

Gross MD. Growth of hyperkinetic children taking methylphenidate, dextroamphetamine, or imipramine/desimpramine. *Pediatrics* 1976; 58: 423–431.

Guilleminault C, Carskadon M, Dement WC. On the treatment of rapid eye movement narcolepsy. *Arch Neurol* 1974; 30: 90–93.

Mendelson WB. Clinical neuropharmacology of sleep. *Clin Neuropharm* 1990; 8: 153–160.

Mendelson WB. Insomnia and related sleep disorders. *Psych Clin N Am* 1993; 16: 841–851.

Mendelson WB. Subjective vs objective tolerance during chronic administration of triazolam. *Clin Drug Invest* 1995; 10: 276–279.

Mendelson WB. Adverse reactions to sedative/hypnotics: three years' experience. *Sleep* 1997; 19: 702–706.

Mendelson WB, Jain, B. An assessment of short-acting hypnotics. *Drug Safety* 1995; 4: 257–270.

Mendelson WB. Neuropharmacology of sleep induction by benzodiazepines. *Crit Rev Neurobiol* 1992; 16: 221–232.

Mendelson WB. The use of sedative/hypnotic medication and its correlation with falling down in the hospital. *Sleep* 1997; 19: 698–701.

Mitler MM, Hajdukovic RM. Relative efficacy of drugs for the treatment of sleepiness in narcolepsy. *Sleep* 1991; 14: 218–220.

Mohler H, Okada, T. Benzodiazepine receptor: demonstration in the central nervous system. *Science* 1977; 198: 849–851.

Monti JM, Attali P, Monti D, et al. Zolpidem and rebound insomnia: a double blind, controlled polysomnographic study in chronic insomniac patients. *Pharmacopsychiat* 1994; 27: 166–175.

Parkes JD, Baraitser M, Marsden CD, Asselman P. Natural history, symptoms and treatment of the narcoleptic syndrome. *Acta Neurol Scand* 1975; 52: 337–353.

Parrino L, Spaggiari MC, Boselli M, Di Giovanni G, Terzano MG. Clinical and polysomnographic effects of trazodone CR in chronic insomnia associated with dysthymia. *Psychopharmacology* 1994; 116: 389–395.

Pascoe PA. Drugs and the sleep-wakefulness continuum. *Pharmac Ther* 1994; 61: 227–236.

Saletu B, Anderer P, Brandstatter N, et al. Insomnia in generalized anxiety disorder: polysomnographic, psychometric and clinical investigations before, during and after therapy with a long-vs a short-half-life benzodiazepine (quazepam versus triazolam). *Neuropsychobiology* 1994; 29: 69–90.

Shindler J, Schachter M, Brincat S, Parkes JD. Amphetamine, mazindol and fencamfamin in narcolepsy. *Br Med J [Clin Res]* 1985; 290: 1167–1170.

Squires RF, Braestrup C. Benzodiazepine receptors in rat brain. *Nature* 1977; 266: 732–734.

SUGGESTED READINGS

Mendelson WB. Clinical neuropharmacology of sleep. *Clin Neuropharm* 1990; 8: 153–160.

Mendelson WB. Insomnia and related sleep disorders. *Psych Clin N Am* 1993; 16: 841–851.

Mitler MM, Aldrich MS, Koob GF, Zarcone VP. Narcolepsy and its treatment with stimulants. *Sleep* 1994; 17: 352–371.

8 Common Sleep Problems in Children

Ronald Dahl

CONTENTS

1. INTRODUCTION

Sleep problems occur frequently in children. Numerous studies have demonstrated that up to 20–30% of children have complaints or difficulties related to sleep that are regarded as significant problems by their families *(1)*. Many of these problems simply fall within the realm of behavioral difficulties and/or bad habits; nonetheless, even minor sleep problems can be a source of distress, conflict, and insufficient sleep for more than one family member. Furthermore, there is increasing evidence that insufficient sleep from any combination of causes can impact negatively on learning, behavior, and emotions. From a clinical perspective, it is essential to understand that, within this wide range of common sleep problems, there are a subset of serious and treatable sleep disorders in children and adolescents. Thus, the primary care clinician must have the requisite knowledge and clinical skills both to manage

From: *Sleep Disorders: Diagnosis and Treatment*
Edited by: J. S. Poceta and M. M. Mitler © Humana Press Inc., Totowa, NJ

effectively common behaviorally based sleep problems and to identify appropriately the children who require further evaluation and treatment.

The treatment of common childhood sleep problems can be an extremely rewarding aspect of clinical practice. Often, simple interventions can resolve negative patterns of behavior that have been causing distress for the entire family. Such interventions can transform an irritable sleep-deprived high-conflict family environment into a more relaxed, positive, and healthy one. Perhaps most importantly, the primary care physician is in a position to emphasize the role of good sleep habits in general preventative health strategies. Knowledge of the role of sleep in healthy development, clinically based family education, and early behavioral interventions can help children establish good sleep/wake habits early in life. As with many areas of health such as nutrition and exercise, establishing good sleep-related habits early in life sets the stage for long-term health.

For the clinician to provide effective prevention, diagnosis, and treatment of sleep problems or appropriate referral for evaluation of more serious disorders, knowledge and clinical skills are needed in four areas:

1. Some understanding of normal sleep physiology and development of sleep patterns.
2. Knowledge of common sleep disorders, including aspects of the etiology, pathophysiology, and differential diagnoses for common symptoms.
3. Clinical skills to assess sleep habits and symptoms necessary to diagnose sleep disorders.
4. Knowledge of the relevant treatment principles—particularly, behavioral interventions.

2. NORMAL SLEEP IN CHILDREN

Normal sleep physiology is discussed in other chapters of this book relevant to adult sleep disorders and includes the basic physiology of REM and non-REM sleep, the context of circadian influences on sleep, and the patterning of sleep-stage changes. In addition to knowledge of adult sleep physiology, however, we will consider below sleep regulation from a developmental perspective from infancy through adolescence.

2.1. Sleep in Infants

In the first few months of life infant sleep is marked by three features:

1. Large amounts of sleep—average sleep durations are about sixteen hours per day in the first month of life.
2. Short bouts of sleep scattered throughout the twenty-four hour period.
3. Onset of sleep beginning with REM sleep, followed by non-REM sleep.

> At six to nine months of age, the particular habits and associations as infants fall asleep at night become a critical step in the development of sleep habits that affect night waking. Learning to fall asleep with minimal parental intervention and without nursing or a bottle helps establish self-comforting behaviors for infants (see text).

During the rest of the lifespan, sleep is entered first through non-REM sleep, except in some disorders, such as narcolepsy.

At about two to three months of age, there are a series of changes in sleep that include the emergence of sleep spindles, delta sleep, and a circadian rhythm in body temperature. By three to six months of age, sleep is beginning to be distributed primarily to the nighttime period with daytime naps becoming consolidated into a more structured time frame. Another transition occurs in the interval from six to nine months of age, when infants begin to be more aware of their external environment and also begin to exhibit more fear behaviors. Older infants become more cognizant of and reactive to the presence or absence of a parent and begin to show separation anxiety and fear of strangers (Box 1).

The most critical issue for most parents of young children is the time of "settling," when infants begin to "sleep through the night." These issues will be addressed further under the topic of infant night-waking; however, the main principle is that infants—even good sleepers—continue to awaken five to eight times a night, usually following normal sleep cycle transitions throughout toddlerhood and childhood. The primary difference between "good sleepers" and "bad sleepers" is whether the infants are able to *put themselves back to sleep* or whether they require parental intervention to do so. The term "self-soothers" has been used to describe the children who are able to return to sleep by themselves in contrast to "signalers" who require parental assistance (e.g., nursing, rocking) to return to sleep. In part, an issue that determines the development of self-soothing versus signaling is the manner in which infant goes to sleep initially, particularly in the period from six to nine months. An infant who usually falls asleep when being nursed, rocked, or with a bottle or a pacifier will often need the same conditions following normal nighttime wakenings (1:00 AM, 3:00 AM, and 5:00 AM, and so on), in order to go back to sleep. Conversely, a self-soothing infant is often able to put him or herself back to sleep following normal middle of the night awakenings without parental involvement, perhaps

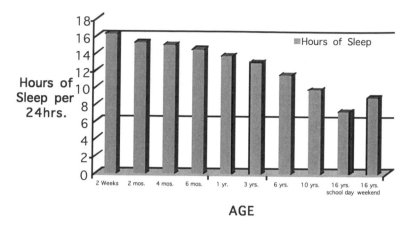

Fig. 1. Developmental changes in sleep duration.

by hugging a stuffed animal, twirling a strand of his or her hair, or thumb sucking. Thus, the parents of a "self-soothers" often perceive that their infant is "sleeping through the night."

Other issues which effect sleep patterns during the first year of life include feeding schedules, colic, medical disorders that can disrupt sleep (e.g., otitis media, atopic dermatitis, or any source of pain or distress), and sleeping arrangements (i.e., cosleeping, family bed, separate room, and so forth) A full discussion of these issues is beyond the scope of this chapter. For further discussion, see refs. *(2,3)*.

2.2. Sleep in Children

During toddler and preschool ages, the amount of sleep continues to decrease (Fig. 1); however, the total amount of sleep required and patterns of daytime naps show large individual differences across toddler and preschool ages. Typically, in the US, naps usually decrease to two per day by fifteen months, one per day by age three years, and most children give up regular napping by five to six years of age.

Across school ages, there is a slight, but steady decrease in the average amount of sleep. The average six- to seven-year-old obtains approximately 10 hours of sleep per night; by the beginning of adolescence, this decreases to about nine hours per night. One other observation about early school age children is their remarkable alertness during the day. School age children are very deep and efficient sleepers yet are very alert (resistant to falling asleep) when they are awake. This pattern appears to change at or near puberty.

> Adolescents physiologically need a great deal of sleep but are often sleep deprived by the combination of late-night activities and early morning school times combined with erratic schedule changes on weekends.

2.3. Sleep in Adolescents

With the onset of adolescence, there are a number of developmental changes in sleep regulation that have been the focus of a great deal of investigation and discussion. These can be broken into three categories:

1. There is an increase in daytime sleepiness—that is, even if adolescents continue to obtain the same amount of sleep as when they were younger, they show more objectively measured daytime sleepiness than prepubertal children.
2. There appears to be a circadian shift near puberty, manifesting as a strong tendency to stay up later at night and to "sleep in" later in the morning.
3. There are enormous social influences further contributing to the tendency to stay up late at night, particularly on weekends.

These three influences converge, contributing to extremely high rates of erratic sleep/wake schedules and daytime sleepiness among adolescents. There is a dramatic discrepancy in adolescence between the amount of sleep obtained on school nights, compared to weekends and vacations. As a result, many adolescents have schedules with late bedtimes and wake-up times on weekends and vacations yet need to get up very early on school days. Rather than shift their circadian systems to the early schedule, many remain "stuck" in an intermediate state, since it can take several days to weeks to completely reset the circadian clock. Many adolescents are severely sleep-deprived on school days, in addition to trying to perform in school at a time when their biological clock is set for sleeping (morning). The combination of sleep deprivation and circadian shifts can lead to profound daytime sleepiness and resulting difficulties with concentration and mood. Large numbers of adolescents fall asleep in school or show other signs of inadequate sleep. The magnitude of these problems appears to be increasing *(4,5)* (Box 2).

3. COMMON SLEEP DISORDERS

3.1. Sleep Problems in Infants and Toddlers

In the first three years of life, the most prevalent difficulty of sleep in most families is difficulty getting the child to go to sleep and stay asleep.

Fifteen to thirty percent of families report significant distress in this area. Difficulties with getting infants and toddlers to sleep through the night are not only a source of sleep disruption for many family members, but they are also a source of conflict and negative emotion among family members that can contribute to negative parent-child interactions, marital discord, and in some cases, child abuse (2).

There are a few important clinical principles relevant to this problem. First, it is easier to prevent than to treat. From six to nine months of age, infants can learn adaptive sleep-onset associations, learning to "self-comfort," as they initially go to sleep. Once children have learned self-comfort to sleep, they are able to repeat the behavior later to return to sleep after brief awakenings at night. Helping an infant learn to fall asleep with minimal parental interaction is a good way to teach this skill at six to nine months.

Once nighttime waking (with parental struggles) has become an established pattern, treating the problem requires a global approach, addressing a variety of social and behavioral issues. Often, there have been months of repeated battles between parents and child about sleeping and waking. This can be very complex area of behavioral pediatrics and has been discussed by numerous clinicians and investigators; an outline to intervention techniques is given in Table 1. A nice summary of this area has been provided by France et al. (2). Approaches to this problem and treatment principles are discussed later in this chapter.

3.2. Cosleeping and the Family Bed

One area of controversy in child-rearing practices is the issue of infants and children cosleeping with a parent and/or the concept of the family bed. Although a full discussion of this is beyond the scope of this chapter, there are a few important points to be made:

1. On the one hand, it is clear that in many cultures, particularly across the scope of human history, cosleeping and family bed sharing have been normative and do not appear to be associated with psychological or physical problems in these contexts.
2. However, it is clear that when children feel physically and emotionally safe, most are quite capable of learning to sleep alone in their own beds and cribs from an early age with no evidence that this creates problems or difficulties for most children. This situation is pragmatic for most families in modern western cultures.
3. Ambivalence and inconsistency regarding the acceptability or practice of cosleeping are a common source of sleep problems in children. Erratic parental rules that sometimes allow the child in the parental bed but sometimes insist the child sleep alone can be confusing to the

Table 1

Advantages, Disadvantages, and Application of Specific Behavioral Treatments for Sleep Problems in Infants and Very Young Children

Technique	Advantages	Disadvantages	Applications	Contraindications
Unmodified systematic ignoring	Rapid. Consistent parental responses promote efficient learning.	Parental resistance and noncompliance. Duration of crying. Spontaneous recovery.	First-time interventions. Motivated parents.	Previous intervention failure. Negative conditioned responses.
Minimal check with systematic ignoring	Rapid. Crying may be of shorter duration. Parent reassured about infant well-being.	Parental presence may trigger intense crying bursts.	First-time interventions. Parents who wish to check the infant.	Previous intervention failure. Negative conditioned responses.
Parental presence with systematic ignoring	Rapid. Less infant crying. Less anticipatory parental anxiety. Parent reassured about infant well-being.	Parental distraction from crying not possible. Parental resistance for practical reasons.	Flexible parents. Parents or infants with separation anxiety.	Parents unable to be in close proximity of their infant without intervening.
Gradual systematic ignoring	Gradual. Parent reassured about infant well-being.	Requires longer-term commitment. Parent must be well organized. Possibility of delayed PERB.[a] Settling problems cannot be handled gradually. More risk of disruptions due to illness.	Healthy infant. Well-organized parents. Anxious parents.	Infants with settling problems. Infants with regular minor illnesses. Parents unable to time and carefully reduce interventions. Cosleeping.
Medication (e.g., chloral hydrate) with systematic ignoring	Relatively rapid. Less infant crying. Less anticipatory parental anxiety.	Parent resistance to medication. Parents less focused on behavior and view the medication as the solution.	Anxious parents. Previous intervention failures. Infants with negative conditioned responses.	None, other than those associated with medication.

[a]PERB, "post-extinction response burst," refers to the burst of unwanted behaviors (in this case, night crying/waking) in the initial period after withdrawing a reinforcer. For example, if parents ignore temper tantrums, there is a burst of worsening tantrums before they go away. Adapted from ref. 2 with permission.

child. Furthermore, some children might get mixed messages from one parent, other family members, or peers about the appropriateness of cosleeping.

Thus, it appears that decisions about cosleeping or family beds are primarily a matter of choice for the individual family with most of the conflicts and difficulties arising from ambiguities or inconsistencies regarding sleep habits, sleep associations, and the appropriateness of sleep arrangements. There are some exceptions to these principles; often, these issues must be considered within a larger framework of the cultural context, individual family situation, and specifics of regarding the child's sleep difficulties (6).

3.3. Common Sleep Disorders in Childhood

Certain common sleep disorders will be discussed together in subsequent sections. Parasomnias are the most common sleep disorder in childhood and include sleep-walking, sleep-talking, night terrors, nightmares, and some bed-wetting. A second common sleep disorder in this age group is insomnia or difficulty in falling asleep. A third common sleep disorder in childhood is obstructive sleep apnea syndrome, which is usually the result of enlarged tonsils and adenoids.

3.4. Common Sleep Disorders in Adolescents

One of the most important disorders related to sleep in adolescents falls into the general category of erratic sleep/wake schedules and delayed sleep-phase syndrome. A tendency to stay up late at night, difficulty falling asleep at earlier bedtimes, and difficulty getting up for school are patterns of sleep habits that are extremely common in teenagers. Shifting to very late schedules on weekends and vacations is a related (and sometimes causal) component of this problem. Although this general pattern is considered to be within the realm of "normal" in many teenage groups, in its severe form, it can result in significant functional impairment, days and weeks of missed school, and have profound effects on mood and behavior. Insufficient and erratic sleep may not only contribute to difficulties with mood, attention, school performance, but many possibly result in alcohol and drug use (4). Finally, teenagers are a very high risk group with regard to automobile accidents, with the majority of fatal accidents occurring between midnight and 5:00 AM—a time when sleepiness is most likely to be high, often in synergy with the effects of alcohol—a lethal combination.

Insomnia also occurs commonly during adolescence and overlaps with anxiety and depressive disorders. It is important to mention that the onset of narcolepsy often begins in late childhood and adolescence.

Narcolepsy is discussed in Chapter 5, and it must be considered in any child or adolescent who demonstrates unexplained daytime sleepiness despite an adequate and undisturbed nighttime sleep in spite of following a stable sleep/wake schedule.

4. COMMON SLEEP COMPLAINTS

Young children don't usually complain directly about their sleep—it is the parents who complain about the sleep of the infants and toddlers. As previously indicated, the primary complaints are that the child doesn't sleep or that he or she sleeps at the wrong time for the parents' schedules. A second point is that young children often show a "paradoxical" reaction when obtaining insufficient or inadequate sleep. That is, sleep-deprived young children (whether from insufficient or disrupted sleep) often look irritable, impulsive, with some symptoms of distractibility and emotional lability, and may seem overly active. The overlap between attention-deficient hyperactivity symptoms and sleep deprivation has been described by numerous clinicians and investigators (1). An important clinical point is that the absence of symptoms of "sleepiness" in a child does not rule out the possibility that a child is receiving insufficient sleep. Parental observations about how tired or "sleepy" toddlers or children appear can be deceptive with respect to their true sleep needs.

Another common parental sleep complaint in children is the occurrence of unusual behaviors in the middle of the night, such as sleepwalking, and night terrors. Night terrors in particular can produce dramatic concerns in parents because the child's appearance is so bizarre during the event: strange facial expressions, appearing awake but acting confused, not recognizing a parent, and occasionally dilated pupils and racing heart. Furthermore, the parent can be distressed by the fact that the child is usually unresponsive to attempts at comforting. Many parents say that children during night terrors look "possessed," a feeling that is further enhanced by the child's lack of memory of the event the following morning. The differential diagnosis and clinical management of these problems is discussed in the section on specific disorders.

4.1. Common Sleep Complaints in Adolescents

By far the most prevalent adolescent sleep complaint is difficulty getting up for school in the morning. Difficulties with daytime sleepiness, tiredness, and irritability are commonly associated with this problem. One of the most important clinical intervention in the adolescent age group is to help the adolescent and his or her family understand the

Table 2
Differential Diagnoses for Sleepiness in an Infant for a Toddler

1. Sleep onset association disorder.
2. Conditioned night feeding or drinking.
3. Colic.
4. Food allergy insomnia.
5. Night-waking associated with medical disorders, pain, and/or discomfort.
6. Separation anxiety disorder.
7. Severe psychosocial stressors.

consequences of the inadequate sleep and late-night schedules that are so frequent.

However, some older children and adolescents complain of insomnia, primarily of the sleep-onset type. There is sometimes an overlap with anxiety and depressive symptoms, and psychiatric disorders must be considered in most adolescents who present a sleep complaint. Caffeine use, erratic schedules, conditioned insomnia, and fears are also of potential importance, as well as the wider range of issues discussed in Chapter 2 on adult insomnia.

It is also important to distinguish between adolescent complaints of lethargy versus sleepiness. That is, although a certain adolescent may complain of difficulty with energy and motivation, he or she might not have difficulty with maintaining wakefulness. "Tiredness," rather than true sleepiness, suggests a alternative differential diagnosis among adolescents.

5. DIFFERENTIAL DIAGNOSES
FOR VARIOUS SLEEP COMPLAINTS

It is clear from the above discussions that there are three main areas of common clinical sleep problems in which it is necessary to consider a differential diagnosis:

1. The infant or toddler with trouble going to sleep and/or with night waking.
2. The child presenting with unusual nighttime behaviors.
3. The tired or sleepy adolescent.

In the infant and toddler age range, there are a wide variety of conditions that can contribute to sleeplessness or night waking. This differential diagnosis is illustrated in Table 2. Over 95% of the clinical cases of the sleepless child can be easily pinpointed with a careful history and physical examination and require no additional clinical testing. For a more comprehensive discussion of the evaluation of infant and toddler sleep problems, see refs. *(2,3,6,7)*.

Table 3
Differential Diagnoses
for Unusual Behaviors in the Middle of the Night

1. Sleep walking.
2. Night terrors.
3. Confusional arousals.
4. Nocturnal seizures.
5. Nightmares (dream anxiety attacks).
6. REM behavior disorder.
7. Waking behaviors.

Table 4
Differential Diagnoses of Sleepiness in the Adolescent

Inadequate amounts of sleep
    Late-night schedules combined with early morning school schedules
    Difficulty falling asleep or night waking (insomnia)
Disturbed nocturnal sleep
    Sleep apnea syndrome
    Frequent nocturnal arousals
    Medical problems disturbing sleep
    Use of drugs and/or alcohol
    Withdrawal from drugs/alcohol
    Restless legs/Periodic limb movement disorder
Increased sleep requirements
    Narcolepsy
    Idiopathic CNS hypersomnolence
    Some cases of depression
    Kleine-Levin Syndrome
Sleep/wake schedule problems
    Erratic sleep/wake schedule
    Circadian and scheduling disorders
    Delayed sleep-phase syndrome

In children age 3–10 years, the most common sleep-related complaint requiring a thorough differential diagnosis is the evaluation of unusual behaviors in the middle of the night. A differential diagnosis for these problems is given in Table 3.

In the adolescent age range, the primary need for differential diagnosis is the evaluation of difficulty waking up for school, and/or daytime sleepiness. The differential diagnosis for this clinical presentation is given in Table 4. A diagnostic algorithm for this presentation is given in Fig. 2 and Table 5 and is discussed at the end of this chapter.

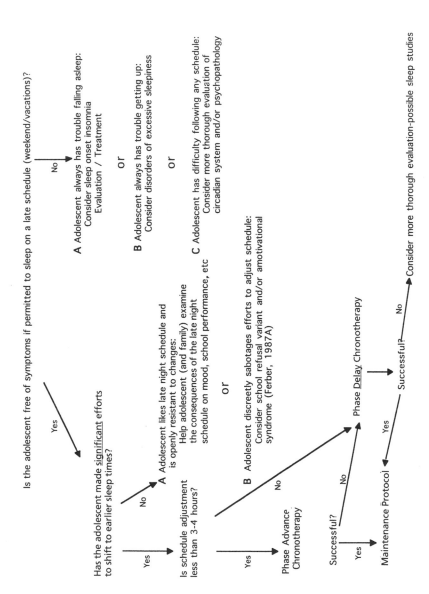

Fig. 2. Evaluation of the adolescent on late-night schedule.

Table 5
Clinical Approach to the Sleepy Adolescent

Carefully collect information on hours in bed, hours asleep, patterns of symptoms, napping, drugs/alcohol/medications, and so forth Examine symptoms when in school and changes on week-ends/vacations.

Adequate number of hours in bed?

Yes		No	
Adequate number of hours asleep?		*Does the sleepiness significantly impact function or mood?*	
Yes	*No*	*Yes*	*No*
1. Symptoms of disrupted sleep? (Snoring, restless sleep, frequent arousals): Evaluation and treatment; may require sleep studies 2. Symptoms of depression? Evaluation and treatment. 3. Symptoms of Kleine–Levin syndrome? Evaluation and treatment. 4. Evidence of drugs/alcohol? Evaluation and treatment. 5. Evidence of objective sleepiness despite adequate night sleep? Consider idiopathic hypersomnolence; may require sleep studies 6. Symptoms of narcolepsy? Refer for sleep consultation and studies.	1. Evidence of delayed sleep-phase insomnia? Consider chronotherapy and bright light therapy. 2. Evidence of depression? Evaluation and treatment. 3. Evidence of drugs or alcohol? Evaluation and treatment. 4. Evidence of conditioned insomnia? Consider behavioral therapy.	What are the specific causes of late night/early morning schedule? Problemsolving with family around specific late-night activities, early rising schedules, erratic sleep/wake hours, and so forth	Recommend increased sleep, good sleep habits

Many young children with disrupted or insufficient sleep may present with symptoms of irritability and poor behavioral control (with some ADHD symptoms) rather than appearing "sleepy."

6. SPECIFIC SLEEP DISORDERS

6.1. Behavioral Problems: Bedtime

The issue of the sleepless infant and toddler has already been addressed. Even in the later preschool ages and school-age children, issues around bedtime behaviors can also be a source of enormous conflict and difficulties in many families. It is important to divide the problem into two components: the child who is resistant to going to bed, and the child who has difficulty falling asleep once in bed.

6.1.1. BEDTIME RESISTANCE

The three most important principles with respect to bedtime resistance are creating an emotional state of calmness and safety, consistent limit setting, and establishing good habits. Bedtime habits should include a wind-down period and a sequence of activities that begin 30–60 minutes before bedtime. Children generally conform well to habitual patterns of behavior once they are established and a key step is to work hard at establishing a comfortable routine that will make bedtime easier to maintain over time. In many households, the "official bedtime" passes with the children engaged in a variety of activities. The parents then begin to provide input at a level of conflict/anger telling the child he or she is late for bed. In some cases, the child has unfinished tasks ranging from homework to tooth brushing. Conflict and yelling at bedtime accompanied by rushing to get last-minute things done are obviously counterproductive to the process of winding down, lowering arousal, and going to sleep. Thus, it requires a fair deal of organization and anticipation to establish positive routines by rewarding the desired behaviors consistently (Box 3).

If a child continues to test limits and not to respond to strategies to reward desirable behaviors, it may become necessary to set consequences for the undesirable behaviors. However, this can still be done within a positive framework to avoid the escalating emotional arousals of yelling, screaming, and flaring tempers. Although the behavioral principles are straightforward, the details as how to help a particular family implement these in specific ways can be challenging.

6.1.2. Difficulty Falling Asleep

One variation of this problem is the child who goes easily to bed but has difficulty falling asleep. Some children repeatedly leave the bed to complain of minor fears, wanting more parental involvement or attention; other children remain quietly in bed but unable to fall asleep. The approach to this problem includes assessing the sources of the child's fears, since fear, distress, or any lack of a sense of safety is antithetical to turning off vigilance at sleep onset. Helping the child feel emotionally and physically safe is often a critical component to this problem. Furthermore, the cognitive processes at bedtime are an important issue. Children often get into the habit of reviewing or replaying memories of stressful events, such as pressing a tongue to a toothache repeatedly—even though it hurts, the behavior is repeated. Children with stressful memories or specific fears can avoid these during the day through distracting activities, but at night, they often ruminate on these thoughts. It is often counterproductive to tell a child to avoid the distressing thoughts, since trying to "not think" about something means that one is actively thinking about it. Instead, help the child actively focus on positive events or images. Depending on the age and inclinations of the child, this can involve creative imagery, self-hypnosis techniques, or systematic relaxation exercises. The principles underlying this intervention are that the parents contribute to an emotional sense of safety, positive emotions, and good associations at bedtime, and the child develops strategies for helping his or her thoughts in the area of positive or neutral events once in bed.

There are overlapping aspects of these two domains—that is, a regular bedtime routine and consistent sequences of steps and habits, such as bedtime story, special quiet time with the parent and pleasant wind-down time, and consistent limits can help a child feel psychologically safe and secure, thus, facilitate going to sleep.

6.2. Parasomnias

Children between the ages of 3 and 10 years of age often demonstrate unusual behaviors in the middle of the night. Sleep-talking, sleep-walking, confusional arousals, night terrors, nightmares, nocturnal seizures, and unusual waking behaviors can all occur in the context of a sudden event erupting from the middle of sleep. Some of the most bizarre and distressing events, such as night terrors, may represent a completely benign entity that responds easily to intervention, whereas a serious abnormality such as nocturnal seizures can sometimes be quite subtle. Therefore, a thorough knowledge of the clinical approach to these problems is extremely important for primary care clinicians.

It is helpful to group these disorders in accordance with the relevant sleep physiology. Beginning with the non-REM parasomnias that appear to be closely related to each other, we will discuss sleep-talking, sleep-walking, confusional arousals, and night terrors. These disorders all occur suddenly out of deep non-REM sleep (stages 3 or 4, or delta) and tend to occur one to two hours after sleep onset. In essence, what happens is that at the end of the first or second sleep cycle, part of the brain attempts to return to light sleep or brief wakefulness, whereas part of the brain remains in deep delta sleep. As the two forces pull against each other, there is sometimes a split—a partial arousal—with part of the brain "awakening" and part of the brain staying deeply asleep. The particular characteristics of the event are highly variable, with some children looking mostly asleep with a few cumbersome awkward movements or sounds, whereas other children will look almost completely awake with agitated rapid movements, wide eyes, dilated pupils, racing heart, sweating, and terrified facial expressions or even blood curdling screams. Events typically last from 15 seconds to a few minutes, then end abruptly with a sudden return to deep sleep. The child sometimes will respond to their parents, but often responses are inconsistent, reflect some confusion, and can be very erratic and unpredictable. Usually, the child has no memory of the events in the morning.

There are three factors which contribute to cause these deep non-REM parasomnias:

1. Family history of similar events.
2. Inadequate sleep from any cause (i.e., overtiredness of any sort increases the likelihood of these events).
3. Emotional state as children fall asleep (falling asleep in an anxious/worried state seems to increase the likeliness of these events).

The classic time for these events to occur is when children give up daytime naps or begin a new school requiring early morning awaking. The combination of stress and change increases the tendency to worry at bedtime, and changes in the sleep/wake schedule (no naps) increase the length of time of wakefulness, increasing the drive to deep delta sleep. Given these interactions, the first interventions are obvious: increasing the total amount of sleep, including regularizing the sleep/wake schedule, and helping children focus on positive thoughts, images, and feelings at bedtime as they fall asleep. It is the experience at our sleep center that over 95% of partial arousals will respond to these two interventions. Furthermore, since these interventions are so benign, they can be implemented as a part of the differential diagnosis. That is, if strange events tend to occur in the first third of the night, are sudden, end

> It is much better to reward positive or desirable behaviors than to punish the undesired behaviors, because conflict tends to increase arousal and interfere with going to sleep.

quickly, the child has no memory of the events, and occur most likely when the child is overly tired, stressed, or worried, it is reasonable to assume that they are parasomnias. Try increasing sleep, regularizing the child's schedule and helping with sleep onset, and see if the events diminish drastically or go away. For further discussion of parasomnias see *(8,9)*.

7. CLINICAL APPROACH TO PARASOMNIAS

As mentioned previously, the most important issue in the clinical assessment of partial arousals from deep sleep is the overall context of the occurrence. Important contextual issues include: the timing of the event (in the first one to three hours of sleep, often like clockwork), the age of the child (the peak age of occurrence for these partial arousals at three to eight years of age), and of a positive family history for sleep-walking or night terrors. Furthermore, if these are occurring in context of being overly tired, stressed, or inadequate sleep, this further supports for the diagnosis of a partial arousal from deep non-REM sleep. Specifically, any difficulty falling asleep, worry at bedtime, or change in schedule such as giving up a nap, waking up early in the morning, or being up late for successive nights increase the likelihood of partial arousal events (Box 4).

The differential diagnosis includes four alternative diagnoses—nightmares, nocturnal seizures, REM behavior disorder, and awake behaviors. Each will be discussed in clinical contrast with night terrors.

7.1. Nightmares

When considering night terrors versus nightmares (also called dream anxiety attacks), remember that nightmares are usually associated with vivid recall of dream content, since they occur during REM sleep. Also, the timing of REM sleep (as indicated earlier) is usually in the second half of the night or last third of the night, as opposed to night terrors, which occur in the first third of the night. Usually, nightmares do not have major motor activity, and there is less anxiety, vocalization, and autonomic discharge during the nightmare. In essence, the child with a nightmare presents to his parents after the nightmare is over, since children are unable to move because of REM-related muscle paralysis during the nightmare. Children often want parental reassurance after a nightmare, are completely awake, afraid, and have trouble going back to sleep. In contrast, night terrors occur when the subject remains partially asleep. Thus, the child usually does not recognize the parents, is not easily reassured or awakened, and the event usually terminates with return to deep sleep with no memory of the event in the morning. Although the distinction between nightmares and night terrors is often straightforward in a school-age child, it can be difficult in a very young toddler with limited verbal abilities.

7.2. Epileptic Seizures

When considering night terrors versus nocturnal seizures, it is valuable to remember that seizures occur predominately during sleep or on arousal from sleep in up to 50% of children with epilepsy. The relationship between sleep and seizures is complex and not well understood. Sleep deprivation appears to increase seizure tendency, sleep onset can precipitated seizures, and the synchronized EEG of Stage 2 sleep appears to facilitate propagation of a seizure focus. Seizures are less likely during Stages 3 and 4 sleep and are much less likely to occur during REM sleep.

There are occasional cases in which seizures occur only during sleep when a seizure disorder has not otherwise been considered. In children with a documented seizure disorder or with a sleep-deprived EEG showing epileptic form discharges, nocturnal seizures must be considered in the differential diagnosis of paroxysmal nocturnal events. For further discussion of this complicated area, please see *(10)*. Obviously, if in doubt, consultation with a pediatric neurologist can be indicated.

7.3. REM Behavior Disorder

REM behavior disorder is theoretically in the differential diagnosis; however, this condition is extremely rare in children and adolescents. REM behavior disorder has been described in adults wherein during REM sleep, the patient moves in a manner suggesting the "acting out" of dream activity. Normally, during REM sleep, there is a dramatic decrease in muscle tone that prevents body movements corresponding to dream activity. A similar pathologic state can be created in animal experiments by small lesions near the locus ceruleus that is believed to be close to the source of motor inhibition during REM sleep. The cases of REM behavior disorder in adult humans have sometimes been associated with lesions in this area or suspected subclinical lesions in this area. There are few convincing reported cases of REM behavior disorder in children. However, this diagnosis should be considered in chil-

> Any source of overtiredness tends to increase the chance of night terrors and sleep-walking events; thus, one should expand the amount of sleep as part of treating these common problems.

dren with any suggestive history or in particular if other central nervous system (CNS) pathology is present or suspected. The timing of the events later in the night when REM is occurring and memory of specific dream imagery corresponding to the actions would suggest the possibility of REM-associated behavior. Treatment approaches are quite different, as this is a very rare and unusual REM-associated movement disorder.

7.4. Waking Behaviors

When evaluating parasomnias that are particularly unusual, consider feigned events in awake children. Occasionally, children may simulate sleep-walking or night terror events when actually being completely awake. The cases we have observed have been in children with previous real sleep-walking or night terror events. In many ways, this is analogous to a child with real seizures or a history of seizures presenting with pseudoseizures. Typically, the child received considerable parental attention following a true partial arousal and subsequently learned to simulate the event before falling asleep at night. In essence, these are learned behaviors that persist in a simulated state, because of some secondary reinforcement or reward the child had received for the behavior. These can usually be differentiated by careful observation and history. In rare cases, sleep studies may be required to convince parents that there is no longer a physiologic basic for the event.

7.5. Treatment Issues

Treatment for partial arousal events needs to focus on the same domains described under the etiology and causal events. Specifically, increasing total amount of sleep, regularizing the sleep/wake schedule, and helping a child focus on positive, relaxing, and comfortable images at sleep onset can all show large positive influences on the frequency of these events (Box 5). It is important to maintain these changes over weeks, and these interventions usually result in a dramatic decrease in the frequency of partial arousal events.

Furthermore, reassurance to the parents of the underlying cause and nature of these events can decrease the overall anxiety and stress in the family. In particular, parents can be instructed to try not to awaken the child and simply help the child go back to sleep or remain in bed. It is important to emphasize physical safety. Although injuries are rare in children during sleep-walking or night terrors, they do occur. Pragmatic steps to insure maximum safety in the physical environment around children with night terrors and sleep-walking needs to be discussed with the family in detail.

Pharmacological therapy can be used, since a wide range of agents (such as benzodiazapines and many antidepressants) are effective at decreasing the rates of these events. However, we have found that pharmacological approaches should be reserved for very severe or unusual partial-arousal events, and such patients should be referred to a pediatric neurologist, psychiatrist, or sleep specialist, if possible. The benzodiazepines have been associated with rebound partial-arousal events if the individual misses a dose or stops the medication.

Other behavioral approaches have included self hypnosis, relaxation exercises, and one novel approach of scheduled awakenings just prior to the time of the usual events. However, other clinicians working within this field have not had as positive response to the scheduled awakenings as the author. (These issues are discussed in more detail in refs. *8,9*.)

7.6. Clinical Approach to the Sleepy Adolescent

Complaints of excessive sleepiness occur frequently in adolescents. A thorough and detailed history is essential to evaluate and to characterize the nature of the sleepiness (that is, fatigue versus inability to stay awake), the frequency and duration of symptoms, and whether the symptoms occur at particular times of day or only in certain situations. A family history of increased sleep needs and sleepiness can be important in the consideration of narcolepsy. Four categories of problems should be considered:

1. Inadequate amounts of sleep.
2. Disturbed nocturnal sleep.
3. Increased sleep requirement despite adequate nocturnal sleep.
4. Circadian and scheduling disorders. The history and evaluation should be directed at characterizing the problem with regard to these categories.

7.7. Inadequate Amounts of Sleep

The most common cause of mild-to-moderate sleepiness in adolescents is an inadequate number of hours in bed. A combination of social schedules leading to late nights with early-morning school requirements

Adolescents with terrible sleep patterns and chronically bad sleep-related habits may require a behavioral contract specifying target behaviors with concrete rewards/punishments for compliance/non-compliance to establish new habits.

can significantly compress the number of hours of sleep. Part-time jobs, sports activities, hobbies, and active social lives can exacerbate this problem. The catch-up sleep of naps, weekends, and holidays can also contribute to the problem by leading to erratic schedules and even later nights. In taking a sleep history, it is important to ask specific questions concerning bedtime schedules. Many families will say the adolescent "usually" goes to bed at a certain time, but when asked for an exact time covering the previous few nights, a much later hour is reported. When assessing the amount of sleep an adolescent is getting, it is important to obtain details of bedtime (such as when the child gets into bed as well as lights-out time), estimates of sleep latency, nighttime arousals, time of getting up in the morning, difficulty getting up, and the frequency, timing, and duration of daytime naps. It is also essential to get details of sleep/wake schedules on weekends, as well as during the school week. When this type of specific information is obtained either by interview or by having the family maintain a sleep diary, evidence of inadequate sleep is often evident. A prospective detailed sleep diary provides the most reliable information.

When inadequate sleep is identified, simply recommending that the adolescent go to bed earlier is not likely to be effective. Often, the primary role of the clinician is to help the entire family understand and acknowledge the consequences resulting from the inadequate sleep. Sleep deprivation frequently contributes to many factors that the family identifies as problems, including falling asleep in school, oversleeping in the morning, fatigue, and irritability. In cases in which the adolescent's school or social functioning is significantly impaired by sleep problems, a strict behavioral contract that is agreed upon by the family can be essential. The contract should specify hours in bed (with only *small* deviations on the weekends) and should target the specific behaviors contributing to bad sleep habits, such as specific late-night activities, erratic napping, or oversleeping for school. The choice of rewards for successes and negative consequences for failures, as well as an accurate method of assessing compliance, are essential components of the contract (Box 6).

7.8. Disturbed Nocturnal Sleep

When symptoms of sleepiness occur despite an adequate schedule of hours in bed, disruptions of sleep should be considered. Disturbances within sleep can be more difficult to assess by history alone. Although some families may describe that the child or adolescent is waking frequently, in other cases, the family may be unaware of subtle disruptions of sleep. The use of drugs or alcohol is an important consideration in these cases. In addition to the obvious effects of late-night stimulants, such as cocaine, there are also more complex drug/sleep interactions. Alcohol, for example, can facilitate sleep onset but can lead to decreased delta and REM sleep. Also, the withdrawal from stimulants, alcohol, and marijuana can produce transient but substantial sleep disruptions. Caffeine is also a commonly used substance in the adolescent population in the form of caffeinated sodas, coffee, and tea. Elimination of caffeine can be an important step in treating symptoms of difficulty falling asleep, which can lead to daytime sleepiness. Prescription medications such as beta-adrenergic agonists for asthma or stimulants for attention-deficit disorder can also result in significant sleep disruptions.

A few specific sources of daytime sleepiness should be considered in this age group: sleep-disordered breathing, narcolepsy, Kleine-Levin Syndrome, and sleep/wake schedule disorders. Sleep apnea and narcolepsy are addressed in Chapters 5 and 6; the approach to these problems in an adolescent is similar to that of an adult.

7.9. Kleine-Levin Syndrome

Symptoms of excessive somnolence, hypersexuality, and compulsive overeating were first described in adolescent boys by Kleine *(11)* and Levin *(12)*. Mental disturbances (irritability, confusion, and occasional auditory or visual hallucinations) have also been reported in these cases.

This syndrome, with over 100 published cases, occurs more frequently in males (3:1) than females. Typically, symptoms begin during adolescence either gradually or abruptly, and in about half the cases, the onset follows a flu-like illness or injury with loss of consciousness. Frequently, there is an episodic nature to the symptoms, with cycles lasting from 1 to 30 days. The syndrome usually disappears spontaneously during late adolescence or early adulthood.

Laboratory tests, imaging studies, EEGs, and endocrine measures do not appear to be helpful in making the specific diagnosis of Kleine-Levin syndrome. It is important to rule out other organic causes of similar symptoms such as a hypothalamic tumor, localized CNS infection, or vascular accident. The presence of neurologic signs, evidence of increased CNS pressure, abnormalities in temperature regulation, abnormalities in water regulation, or other endocrine abnormalities point to an organically based abnormality. A family history of bipolar illness or other signs suggesting an early-onset bipolar illness should also be considered in the differential.

Although stimulant medication or use of lithium carbonate has been reported to be helpful in individual cases, there is no clear consensus on treatment.

7.10. Circadian and Scheduling Disorders

The most common specific problem with this system that is relevant to adolescents is delayed sleep-phase syndrome (DSPS). DSPS often begins with a tendency to stay up late at night, sleeping in late, and/or taking a late afternoon nap. This process often begins on weekends, holidays, or summer vacations. Problems become apparent when school schedules result in morning wake-up battles and difficulties in getting to school. Often, these adolescents cope by taking afternoon naps and getting catch-up sleep on the weekends. Although some of these behaviors occur in many normal adolescents, in extreme cases, the circadian system can become set to such a late time that even highly motivated adolescents can have difficulty shifting their sleep back to an earlier time. In some instances, the attempts by the adolescents (and their families) to correct the problem go against circadian principles. For example, an adolescent who has been going to bed at 3 AM and getting up at noon during a vacation tries to go bed at 10 PM the Sunday night before the first day back at school finds that her physiology is quite resistant to sleep. For a few days, she manages to get up for school by overriding the system (despite inadequate sleep) but then takes a long nap after school. Despite numerous nights of trying to go to bed at 10 PM she is unable to shift her temperature cycle and circadian system back to an earlier phase (Fig. 2, Tables 4 and 5).

The treatment of DSPS consists of two parts. The first is to *gradually* align the sleep system to the desirable schedule. The second is to maintain that alignment. The process of alignment consists of gradual consistent advances in bedtime and wake-up time (15 minutes/day). It is often best to begin from the time the adolescent usually goes to sleep without difficulty. It is important during this process to avoid any naps and to be consistent across weekends and holidays. In severe cases, some adolescents on very late schedules respond more favorably to going around the clock with successive delays in bedtime. This process has been described as phase delay "chronotherapy." Because the biologic clock tends to run on a 25-hour cycle, it accommodates phase delays more easily than phase advances. Hence, the schedule changes can proceed with larger (two to three hour) delays per day. An example is described for an adolescent who has been falling asleep at 3 AM and getting up at noon. On day 1, he stays up until 6 AM then sleeps until 3 PM. On day 2, he goes to bed at 9 AM and sleeps until 6 PM. On day 3, he sleeps from noon until 9 PM; day 4, from 3 PM until midnight; day 5, from 6 PM until 3 AM; day 6 from 9 PM until 6 AM; and day 7, from 10 PM until 7 AM. It is important that the adolescent take no naps during the chronotherapy. Upon waking up, he or she should be active and, if possible during the day, have bright light exposure, such as walking outdoors. Although many adolescents do very well with this type of phase-delay chronotherapy, the first weekend or vacation of returning to old habits can undo a lot of hard work. Particularly in the first two to three weeks following chronotherapy, rigid requirements should be set about wake-up time. Maintenance of the new circadian phase is based on the same principles but usually can be somewhat less rigorous. For example, if the adolescent wants to stay up late on an occasional weekend night, he may be able to do so but should not be permitted to sleep more than one or two hours later than his usual wake-up time for school. Strict behavioral contracts worked out with the parents, having specific rewards for success and serious consequences for failures are essential in this type of intervention.

The use of bright light therapy for circadian rhythm shifting in adults is described by Dr. Kripke in Chapter 3. The same timing and principles of these recommendations are also true for adolescents and can supplement the schedule shifts described above. The use of bright light therapy in the mornings in addition to small phase advances has largely supplanted the need for chronotherapy as treatment of DSPS.

The use of melatonin has also been suggested as a potential treatment for this problem. Currently, there are some preliminary data supporting the use of low-dose melatonin in the evening to assist with the resetting of the timing of sleep to an earlier phase. In some ways, melatonin appears to act as "chemical darkness" to offset the effects of late-night artificial lights in influencing the biological clock. It is important to note the lack of any safety data regarding melatonin use in adolescents. Others have argued that direct control over exposure to light (darkness in the evening and bright light exposure on awakening) can be more effective than melatonin.

At least two other disorders can mimic DSPS. One disorder involves adolescents who appear to have trouble following an early schedule but are not particularly troubled by their late schedule. These adolescents are not motivated to correct the problem, are not particularly troubled by their recurrent experiences of being late for or missing school, and do not show great motivation to change their late-night habits. These adolescents are essentially choosing a late-night schedule. Unless the clinician is able to alter the larger realm of priorities and motivators, these adolescents are very unlikely to respond to any treatment of a sleep/schedule problem.

A second group of adolescents who initially appear to have DSPS reveals a history of requiring very long periods of time to fall asleep, no matter how late they go to bed. In these adolescents, a conditioned insomnia—similar to descriptions in Chapter 2 on adult insomnia—is a larger component of the problem than the schedule itself. For an overview of the clinical approach to the adolescent with DSPS, see Fig. 2.

8. CONCLUSION

In closing, it is important to reemphasize the overlap of a majority of sleep problems in children and adolescents with behavioral/emotional problems in these age groups. Clearly, there are bidirectional effects; sleep disturbances are capable of causing behavioral/emotional changes as well as vice versa. From a clinical perspective, the overlap and interaction between sleep regulation and behavioral/emotional problems creates a complex situation. The interested reader is referred to a recent volume that addresses many aspects of these interactions *(1)*.

REFERENCES

1. Dahl RE. Child and adolescent sleep disorders, in *Child and Adolescent Clinics of North America* (Dahl RE., ed.), W. B. Saunders, Philadelphia, 1996, p. 3.
2. France KG, Henderson J, Hudon SM. Fact, act, and tact: A three-stage approach to treating the sleep problems of infants and young children, in *Child and Adolescent Clinics of North America* (Dahl RE., ed.), W. B. Saunders, Philadelphia, 1996, pp. 581–600.
3. Anders TF, Halpern LF, Hua J. Sleeping through the night: a developmental perspective. *Pediatrics* 1992; 90: 554–560.
4. Carskadon MA. Adolescent sleepiness: increased risk in a high-risk population. *Alcohol, Drugs, Driving* 1990; 6:3: 317–328.
5. Dahl RE. Sleep in behavioral and emotional disorders, in *Principles and Practice of Sleep Medicine in the Child*, 2nd ed., vol. 2 (Kryger M, Roth T, Dement W, eds.), W. B. Saunders Company, Philadelphia, 1995, pp. 147–153.
6. Wolfson AR. Sleeping patterns of children and adolescents: Developmental trends, disruptions and adaptations, in *Child and Adolescent Psychiatric Clinics of North America* (Dahl RE, ed.), W. B. Saunders, Philadelphia, 1996, pp. 549–568.
7. Ferber R. Sleeplessness in the child, in *Principles and Practice of Sleep Medicine* (Kryger M, Roth M, Dement T, Dement WC, eds.), W. B. Saunders, Philadelphia, 1989, pp. 633–639.

8. Rosen GM, Ferber R, Mahowald MW. Evaluation of Parasomnias in children, in *Child and Adolescent Psychiatric Clinics of North America* (Dahl RE, ed.), W. B. Saunders, Philadelphia, 1996, pp. 601–616.

9. Dahl RE. Parasomnias, in *Handbook of Prescriptive Treatments for Children and Adolescents* (Ammerman RT, Last CG, Hersen M, eds.), Allyn and Bacon, Boston, MA, 1994, pp. 281–299.

10. Brown LW. Sleep and epilepsy, in *Child and Adolescent Psychiatric Clinics of North America* (Dahl RE, ed.), W. B. Saunders, Philadelphia, 1996, pp. 701–714.

11. Kleine. Periodische schlafsucht. *Monatsschr Psychiatr Neurol* 1925; 57: 285.

12. Levin M. Narcolepsy and other varieties of morbid somnolence. *Arch Neurol Psychiatry* 1929; 22: 1172.

Sleep Disorders in Primary Care Practice

Richard D. Simon, Jr., Eric M. Ball, and Jennings C. Falcon II

1. INTRODUCTION

In 1991, the National Commission on Sleep Disorders Research, composed of the nation's premier sleep medicine specialists and chaired by Dr. William Dement of Stanford University, found that 40 million Americans were ill with various sleep disorders *(1)*, the majority of whom were not diagnosed, thus, not treated. Despite the existence of a large body of sleep medicine science and the availability of effective treatment for most sleep disorders, this knowledge base was virtually absent among primary care physicians and the lay public. After reviewing the computerized records of 10 million patients in large primary care databases, the Commission found only 73 diagnoses of obstructive sleep apnea (OSA), whereas thousands of cases would have been expected, based on known prevalence figures. In a survey of all accredited

From: *Sleep Disorders: Diagnosis and Treatment*
Edited by: J. S. Poceta and M. M. Mitler © Humana Press Inc., Totowa, NJ

U.S. medical schools, the amount of time spent teaching medical students about sleep medicine was less than two hours *(2)*. Thus, primary care health care providers were woefully undertrained to diagnose and treat the millions of patients in the US who are afflicted with sleep disorders. The Commission recommended that a nationwide program be instituted to educate the general population and the medical profession about sleep.

2. CONCEPT AND IMPLEMENTATION OF THE WALLA WALLA PROJECT

It was from these recommendations and findings that the Walla Walla Project was started by William Dement of Stanford University and German Nino-Murcia of the Sleep Medicine and Neuroscience Institute in Palo Alto. The purpose of this demonstration project was to bring the diagnosis and treatment of sleep disorders medicine into primary care practice by teaching a group of primary care physicians about sleep medicine and providing these physicians with the technical expertise to diagnose and treat sleep-disordered patients.

Walla Walla was an ideal community for such a project. At the time of the conception of the Walla Walla Project in late 1991, the nearest certified sleep centers (Portland, OR and Seattle, WA) were 250 miles away as Walla Walla is a rural community, located in southeastern Washington. Its population was 26,748, and the population of Walla Walla County was 48,439. This community has three hospitals: St. Mary Medical Center, Walla Walla General Hospital, and the Walla Walla Veterans Administration Hospital, totaling approximately 300 beds. Approximately 100 physicians practiced in this community in 1991, 31 of whom practiced at the multispecialty Walla Walla Clinic.

Physicians of the Walla Walla Clinic were approached by Drs. Dement and Nino-Murcia, and it was agreed to initiate the Walla Walla Project. Prior to any educational intervention, 752 randomly selected primary care records were reviewed; a primary sleep-related condition was suspected in six. One had nocturnal oximetry done, and two were referred for sleep medicine consultations. Thus, physicians at the Walla Walla Clinic were not diagnosing or treating sleep disorders to any significant degree prior to the start of the Walla Walla Project.

A respiratory therapist from the Walla Walla Clinic went to Palo Alto, where he trained in polysomnographic technology. Drs. Dement and Nino-Murcia then came to Walla Walla and presented a weekend course on sleep medicine to interested physicians. Among those in attendance were the three authors (RDS, EMB, general internists; JCF, neurologist) and numerous other physicians from a variety of specialties, including internal medicine, pediatrics, radiology, gastroenterology, and otolaryngology. Physicians then began to ask their patients about sleep and to study appropriate patients. When indicated, 16 channel computerized polysomnography was performed, initially in the patients' homes. Nocturnal positive airway pressure titrations were performed at the Walla Walla Clinic with a technologist in attendance. Data disks were sent to Palo Alto for scoring and returned to Walla Walla for interpretation. Weekly telephone conferences were conducted between the Walla Walla team and Dr. Nino-Murcia. Since summer 1993, all diagnostic studies were performed at the Walla Walla Clinic Sleep Laboratory, attended by a technologist. Later in 1993, a split-night polysomnogram/positive airway pressure titration protocol was instituted in an effort to diagnose and treat patients with severe OSA in a more cost-effective manner.

During the first two years of the project, the authors attended numerous other continuing medical education (CME) offerings in sleep medicine. In March 1994, the authors started scoring and interpreting all sleep studies locally. Periodic sleep meetings are still held locally to discuss interesting and difficult cases. In December 1994, the Walla Walla Clinic moved its sleep laboratory to St. Mary Medical Center, and the Kathryn Severyns Dement Sleep Disorders Center was founded and named in honor of Dr. Dement's mother, who had been a lifelong resident of Walla Walla prior to her death in 1994 at the age of 104. The sleep center is currently in the process of applying for Sleep Center Certification by the American Sleep Disorders Association.

3. SLEEP DISORDERS IN WALLA WALLA

During the first two years of the Walla Walla Project, a large number of patients were diagnosed with significant sleep disorders (3). Three hundred and sixty patients were studied with polysomnography (Table 1). The vast majority of patients studied had OSA (77%) and were treated with positive airway pressure devices (either continuous positive airway pressure [CPAP] or bilevel positive airway pressure [BiPAP]). By patient report, compliance rates of CPAP/BiPAP usage were similar to rates seen at established sleep centers. A large number of patients (18%) were found to have periodic limb movements of sleep (PLMS), often in association with OSA. Significant numbers of patients were found to have circadian rhythm disturbances (5%) and inadequate sleep hygiene (8%). Narcolepsy was diagnosed in 0.6% of the patients studied. During this period, patients diagnosed with sleep disorders had an average of 2.2 studies per patient.

Table 1
Summary of Sleep Diagnoses
in 360 Patients Studied with Polysomnography
Between March 1992–February 1994[a]

Diagnosis	Percentage affected
OSA	77
UARS	5
PLMS	18
Narcolepsy	0.6
Sleep hygiene	8
Circadian	5
Other	15

[a]Some patients have more than one diagnosis.

Table 2
Sleep Diagnoses in 597 Patients
from March 1994–February 1996

Diagnosis	Percentage affected
OSA	83
UARS	4
PLMS (primary diagnosis)	3
Miscellaneous	4
Incomplete data	6

Of the patients studied during the first two years, 82% derived their primary care from the Walla Walla Clinic, and only 4% were referred from outside of the Walla Walla area. A large percentage of the patients came from the primary care practices of two of the authors (RDS, EMB). Twenty-six percent of all patients were diagnosed and directly managed by their primary care physician, without consultation from one of the authors. As the authors developed more expertise in sleep medicine, their primary care colleagues increasingly referred patients for consultation rather than directly for sleep laboratory testing. Notably, within the first two years of the Walla Walla Project, the diagnosis and treatment of patients with sleep disorders by all Walla Walla Clinic physicians increased substantially.

From March 1994, when the authors began scoring and interpreting all of the polysomnograms locally, to March 1996, 597 individual patients were studied with polysomnography (Table 2). Eight hundred and eighty-five polysomnograms, split-night studies, and titration stud-

Table 3

Walla Walla Clinic Primary Care Internists Requesting
Polysomnograms/Titration Studies Between March 1994–February 1996[a]

Primary care MD	Patients without consult	Patients with consult
RDS	217	1
EMB	87	0
Internist 1	19	6
Internist 2	9	22
Internist 3	7	9
Internist 4	9	46

[a]No consult means that the primary care physicians managed the patients entirely alone. Consult means that sleep consultation was obtained either before the study or after it had been completed. RDS and EMB are authors.

Key points:

- The diagnosis and treatment of sleep disorders at the Walla Walla Clinic grew markedly from 1991 to 1996.
- Sleep disorders interacted with many common conditions such as headache, hypertension, and stroke.
- Large numbers of patients with previously unrecognized sleep disorders were able to reduce personal suffering and improve their health.

---

ies were performed. Ninety-nine Multiple Sleep Latency Tests (MSLTs) were performed. The average number of studies per patient dropped from 2.2 during the previous two years to 1.7, largely as a result of the institution of a split-night protocol for the diagnosis and treatment of severe OSA. During this period, the most common diagnosis remained OSA (83%). Once again, the majority of patients came from the practices of two of the authors (Table 3). The diagnosis and treatment of sleep disorders by other internists at the Walla Walla Clinic were variable. Most of the other internists diagnosed fewer patients, which possibly reflects less aggressive questioning of patients about sleep issues than was the case with the authors. Some preferred to manage their own patients, and some preferred to refer the majority of their sleep-disordered patients to the authors.

The percentage of patients undergoing polysomnography who were also referred for sleep medicine consultation increased from 44% in the period of 1992–1994 to 65% in the period of 1994–1996. The reasons

Table 4
Sleep Diagnoses in 857 Established Patients
(first seen before 1992) Who Have Been Seen Since 1992
in One of the Author's (RDS) Primary Care Practice

Diagnoses	Percentage of sleep diagnoses	Percentage of total practice
OSA	61	8.5
PLMS	12	1.6
Primary snoring	6.7	1
Shiftwork	2.5	
Advanced sleep-phase syndrome	1.7	
Delayed sleep-phase syndrome	0.8	
Others	15.3	

There are 119 patients who have had sleep diagnoses made since 1992. Percentages are of those with sleep diagnoses. Percentages in parenthesis indicate total percentages in the primary care practice. The "others" category includes insomnia, narcolepsy, parasomnias, insomnia secondary to medical conditions, etc.

for this are multifactorial and include recognition of expertise of the authors, the variety of sleep laboratory testing options, and the internal policy requirement that a sufficient history and physical exam be done prior to ordering a sleep study.

4. EXPERIENCE OF ONE OF THE AUTHORS (RDS)

The experience of one of the authors provides a deeper understanding of the scope of sleep disorders in primary care. At the start of the project, he had a full primary care practice, but as his experience in sleep medicine grew, so did the number of sleep consultations, such that currently 80% of his practice is currently devoted to sleep medicine. In April 1996, he became a Diplomate of the American Board of Sleep Medicine. Thus from the start of the Walla Walla Project in 1992 until 1996, his practice has evolved from a primary care internal medicine practice into a subspecialty sleep medicine practice.

Computerized records of his practice have been kept since 1984. From these records, a total of 857 patients were identified who had established primary care with RDS prior to the start of the Walla Walla Project and were seen in his practice at least once since 1992. Of these patients, 119 (14%) have significant sleep disorders (Table 4). Many of the patients were identified by routinely incorporating sleep questions in the review of systems conducted during routine visits, rather than by waiting for spontaneous patient complaints of daytime sleepiness, dis-

Table 5
Number of Sleep Medicine Consultations
from February 1992 through October 1996
of One of the Authors (RDS)

Year	Number of consultations
1992	16
1993	98
1994	118
1995	177
1996 (10/31/96)	179

Table 6
Sleep Diagnosis of Consultations
in One of the Author's (RDS) Sleep Medicine Practice[a]

Diagnosis	Percentage
OSA	71
PLMS/RLS	12
Narcolepsy	4
Delayed sleep-phase syndrome	5.9
Advanced sleep-phase syndrome	0.4
Insomnia	7.9
Primary snoring	5.5
Others	9.6

[a]Some patients have more than one diagnosis.

rupted nocturnal sleep, snoring, or abnormal sleep behaviors. Of the patients with sleep disorders, most have OSA (61%) although a significant number have PLMS (12%). Thus, 8.5% of the patients in RDS's primary care practice have OSA, the vast majority of whom are being treated with positive airway pressure devices.

Additionally, this author's sleep medicine consultative practice grew sequentially each year since the start of the Walla Walla Project (Table 5). The majority of cases continued to be referred for OSA (71%) and PLMS (12%) although significant numbers of patients were seen for circadian rhythm abnormalities and insomnia (Table 6).

5. EDUCATIONAL EFFORTS

The authors have provided over 30 hours CME 1 opportunities to health care providers, locally and regionally, as well as numerous hours of non-CME education to health care providers and the general public.

Health care providers are encouraged to incorporate a group of sleep medicine questions in the general review of systems. The major determinants of sleep and factors that modify sleep are taught to local health care providers. Health care providers are encouraged to take complaints of sleepiness, fatigue, snoring, and disturbed sleep seriously and to complete a sleep history from patients with these complaints. Health care providers are taught to warn patients of the dangers of trying to function with a large sleep debt.

As a result of the Walla Walla Project, health care providers in Walla Walla have been equipped with more information and techniques with which to improve the lives of their patients. The following cases illustrate these points.

5.1. Case 1

An eight-year-old female has been in good health until recently; her parents divorced one year earlier and she developed abdominal pain at night. Her weight has remained normal and she has no vomiting, diarrhea, fevers, chills, or sweats. Her pediatrician suspects stress-induced gastritis and provides for appropriate counseling. Over the next several weeks, her abdominal discomfort resolves; however, her mother requests another appointment because the patient has now developed insomnia. The pediatrician inquires about bedtime and wake time on school days and on weekends. On school days, the patient goes to bed at 9 PM but can't fall asleep. She demands attention from her mother and often cries if she doesn't get it. She finally falls asleep by midnight. Her mother finds it impossible to awaken her at 6:30 AM in time for school, so the child is often late to school. On weekends, the mother allows the child to go to bed at midnight, at which time the child does not have difficulty falling asleep. She typically sleeps in until 10–11 AM on weekends. Although the pediatrician believes that unresolved stress over the divorce is still problematic, he strongly suspects the sleep complaints are those of DSPS. He advises that she sleep on the east side of the house with her shades open and that she awaken every day at 6:30 AM and get as much sunlight as possible for 45–60 min. She may sleep in only until 7–8 AM on weekends and is to get bright light immediately upon awakening. She is to go to bed at night only when sleepy. Within two weeks, she is going to bed and to sleep at 9 PM and awakening, alert, at 6:30 AM.

5.1.1. Discussion

This patient's sleep was probably initially disrupted by the stress of her parents divorce. During this time, she developed a pattern of going to bed later at night and of sleeping later in the morning. The pediatrician appropriately diagnosed adjustment disorder and provided adequate counseling. However, the child's sleep complaints persisted. Because of the Walla Walla Project and its education of physicians, the pediatrician recognized that persistent evening insomnia and morning sleepiness were the hallmarks of DSPS, which he correctly treated by focusing on a consistent wake-up time with bright light, and recommending bedtime only when the child was sleepy.

5.2. Case 2

A 48-year-old man with labile unmedicated hypertension was referred by his family practitioner for neurology consultation to assess his incapacitating headaches, previously minimally responsive to conventional over-the-counter (OTC) and prescription analgesics plus chiropractic intervention. At the time of consultation, he had been experiencing headaches for only the previous year. Their frequency was estimated as 1–3 per week; their duration ranged from 6–24 hours and were typically 9 hours. They fulfilled criteria for migraine headache without aura and were described as always commencing out of nocturnal sleep. His daughter additionally had less frequent migraine headaches with and without aura.

Because of his body habitus (body mass index [BMI], 42.2 and neck circumference, 21 inches) careful inquiry was directed towards the possibility of OSA, but the patient and his wife denied relevant symptoms other than simple snoring to support this speculation.

Over the ensuing year, the patient was successfully treated with oral antimigraine rescue pharmacotherapy and preventive pharmacotherapy with long-acting propranolol that additionally rendered him normotensive. He was seen on eight follow-up visits over the next year, by which time he commented on being "tired" but didn't believe himself to be "sleepy," because he could stay awake in the daytime, if he tried. His wife noted "breathing irregularity" during his sleep. He was experiencing one headache per month warranting rescue treatment plus once-weekly brief mild headaches.

At this time, the suspicion of OSA was high enough that the patient agreed to overnight nocturnal polysomnography and next day MSLT. Nocturnal polysomnography demonstrated severe OSA with a respiratory disturbance index (RDI) of 94 (apnea index, 28, hypopnea index, 66 these numbers represent events per hour of sleep) and a nadir oxygen saturation of 67%. MSLT demonstrated severe sleepiness (mean sleep latency, 1.9 minutes). BiPAP titration was performed, normalizing his RDI at 4.

Following treatment with BiPAP, the patient's wife repeatedly remarked "he has more energy and is more alert." The patient was "astounded by the lack of any headaches," which prompted a successful taper off of propranolol. At last contact, three years after implementation and with 100% compliance with BiPAP therapy, the patient remains completely free of headaches. He enjoys a great deal more energy, and he does not fall asleep under any circumstance in the daytime.

5.2.1. DISCUSSION

This patient was referred to one of the authors (JCF) for treatment of migraine headaches. Because the patient was obese and had a very large neck, he was carefully questioned about symptoms of OSA, which he and his wife denied. It took several more visits over the next year before the consultant could convince the patient to undergo sleep testing. Sleep laboratory testing confirmed the diagnosis of OSA, and the patient was successfully treated with BiPAP with resolution of his headaches and improvement in his daytime energy level. This case demonstrates that sleep disorders permeate subspecialty medicine in addition to primary care medicine and that knowledge of sleep disorders helps the specialist to identify underlying sleep disorders that can be the precipitating triggers to a multitude of other conditions.

5.3. Case 3

A 72-year-old female primary care patient had requested codeine and other opiate analgesics for a variety of pain conditions for years. Over a decade ago, her previous primary care physician prescribed opiates to treat low back pain. Currently, she complained of nonspecific abdominal pain, and she was found to have a small umbilical hernia that was repaired. She continued to request opiates for persisting abdominal pain without an identifiable cause. When her requests were denied, she complained bitterly of not feeling well and of hurting all over. The patient was an active woman who enjoyed golfing, walking, and exercising at the YMCA frequently. Interestingly, her pain did not interrupt her exercising, and she did not require opiates when she was active. She required opiates only at night or if she was inactive for long periods of time during the day. On careful questioning she admitted to having "weird" dysesthetic sensations in her legs and arms when she went to bed at night. Upon lying down at night she routinely developed an unpleasant sense of restlessness in her legs. She often awakened in order to rub her legs vigorously or to walk around her bed to relieve these symptoms. Her husband remarked that her legs often twitched at night when she slept.

A diagnosis of restless legs syndrome (RLS) was entertained, and therapy with pergolide was instituted. Nocturnal sleep improved, and her symptoms resolved. Her need for opiates lessened, although on occasions she still required codeine, in addition to pergolide, at night to help her sleep. Polysomnography was not performed in this case.

5.3.1. Discussion

This is a case of an elderly woman with chronic use of opiates which were required for treatment of previously unrecognized RLS. By having a high index of suspicion and knowledge of sleep disorders, her primary care provider rendered a proper diagnosis, legitimized her valid long-term requests for opiates, and administered additional appropriate therapy.

These three cases serve to illustrate the manner in which many patients with sleep disorders present to health care providers. The symptoms are often not obviously related to sleep and often suggest other diagnoses (adjustment disorder in Case 1 and drug-seeking behavior in Case 3). Additionally, the course of other medical diseases can be altered by the presence of primary sleep disorders (Case 2, OSA triggering migraine headaches). Because sleep disorders are common, one must always inquire about sleep habits of any patients (Case 1, markedly different sleep hours during school days versus weekends; Case 3, need for opiates, primarily at night) and one must be aware of typical physical exam findings (Case 2, large neck, obesity, coexisting hypertension), which suggest possible sleep disorders. It is unlikely that any of these three patients would have been correctly diagnosed prior to implementation of the Walla Walla Project.

6. CONCLUSIONS

Sleep disorders are among the most common of all medical problems and are present in significant numbers in primary care and subspecialty practices. Sleep disorders can present as isolated disorders, or they can coexist with diseases such as adjustment disorder, headaches, hypertension, myocardial infarction, stroke, and other medical and surgical disorders. Results of the Walla Walla Project support the conclusion of the National Commission on Sleep Disorders Research shows that there are enormous numbers of patients with sleep disorders who are seen every day by primary care and subspecialty providers and who are in need of treatment. Health care providers can begin to diagnose and treat patients with sleep disorders by taking a sleep history that can easily be incorporated into the routine review of systems.

Because of the countless injuries, personal suffering, and even death that results from unrecognized and untreated sleep disorders, health care providers have a responsibility to become knowledgable about sleep and sleep disorders *(4)*. The Walla Walla Project suggests that, with proper supervision and training, health care providers can learn to diagnose and effectively treat patients with sleep disorders. This project also clearly demonstrates the large numbers of patients with unrecognized sleep disorders that are present in primary care medicine and supports the need for better medical education and training in the diagnosis and management of patients with sleep disorders.

REFERENCES

1. National Commission on Sleep Disorders Research Report. Executive summary and executive report, vol. 1. National Institutes of Health, Bethesda, MD, 1993.
2. Rosen C, Rosekind M, Rosevear C, Cole, WE, Dement, WC. Physician Education in Sleep and Sleep Disorders: A National Survey of U.S. Medical Schools. *Sleep* 1993; 16: 249–254.
3. Ball EM, Simon RD, Tall AA, Banks MB, Nino-Murcia G, Dement WC. Diagnosis and treatment of sleep apnea within the community: the Walla Walla Project. *Arch Int Med* 1997; 157: 419–424.
4. Dement WC, Mitler M. It's time to wake up to the importance of sleep disorders. *JAMA* 1993; 269: 1548–1550.

10 Sleep Medicine as Preventive Medicine
Managed Care, Technology, and Outcomes

Stephen F. Johnson

CONTENTS

1. INTRODUCTION

Reflect for a moment about what you have read so far. Millions of people have complaints about the quality and quantity of their sleep. Of 20 patients in your waiting room today, two have significant insomnia, two regularly become sleep-deprived, and one or two have obstructive sleep apnea (OSA). Only one of these patients, or an accompanying family member, will bring the sleep problem to your attention.

Direct interrogation is needed to detect your patients' sleep problems. Before reading this book, you would not have questioned your patients about sleep. You would have missed the chance to help five of

From: *Sleep Disorders: Diagnosis and Treatment*
Edited by: J. S. Poceta and M. M. Mitler © Humana Press Inc., Totowa, NJ

the six patients with sleep disorders in your waiting room. And in the past, you might have been frustrated by the sixth patient—the insomniac—who did speak up. Your conditioned response to the complaint of sleeplessness—a prescription for a sleeping pill—merely brushed the insomniac aside. By overlooking sleep disorders, you missed the chance to make a difference in your patients' lives. Considering the notable efforts you made to treat other common illnesses, why were sleep complaints passed over?

2. WHY PHYSICIANS SHORT-CHANGE SLEEP MEDICINE

Lack of instruction about sleep disorders in medical school and in postgraduate training means that the majority of physicians never learn important facts about sleep medicine. At most, students receive a few perfunctory lectures on sleep and hypnotic medications during medical school. In residency training, the subject of sleep is ignored. Except for the routine "laxative" and "sleeper" orders for patients admitted to the hospital, sleep disorders get little notice either on ward rounds or in the outpatient clinic.

Lack of formal training is not the only reason physicians often overlook sleep disorders. Sleep itself is in short supply for young physicians in their formative years. Staying up late to cram for examinations in medical school is followed by prolonged stints at the hospital, during which the only chance to interview the patient or to study may be late at night. That residents fall asleep quickly whenever a quiet moment presents itself is not a virtuoso skill; rather, a short sleep latency is a sign of insufficient sleep. Nevertheless, many physicians emerge from their postgraduate training with the attitude that sleep is a handicap to be overcome, rather than an indispensable biological function.

The Epworth Sleepiness Scale (ESS) can demonstrate the sleep-deprived state of patients as well as physicians. The ESS is described and shown in Chapter 1. Shown in Fig. 1 are ESS scores for normal subjects, medical students, practicing physicians, sleep apneics, and insomniacs. Medical students have a higher mean and a wider distribution than normal subjects, most probably because of varying degrees of and sensitivity to sleep deprivation. Practicing physicians are closer to normal than medical students, but at least 20% of nonsnoring practicing physicians appear to have excessive daytime sleepiness. As another measure of sleep deprivation, over 50% of practicing physicians report sleeping in an hour or more extra on weekend or vacation days, compared to work days. There are no ESS surveys of resident physicians, but this group almost certainly have a higher degree of sleep deprivation

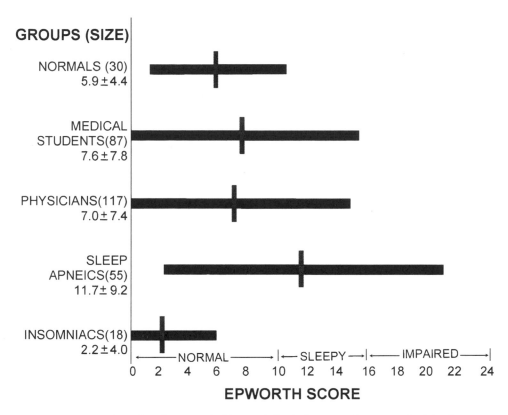

Fig. 1. Daytime sleepiness on the Epworth Scale (mean and two standard deviations). The data on normal subjects, medical students, patients with sleep apnea, and insomniacs were published by M. W. Johns in a series of articles, the most recent of which is cited in the reference section at the end of this chapter. The data on practicing physicians were collected by the author for this chapter and have not been published elsewhere.

than medical students. Take the ESS yourself; how does your own score compare with the various groups in Fig. 1?

Are you still skeptical about the importance of sleep deprivation? Consider the research that has been done on the consequences of lack of sleep among resident physicians, summarized in Table 1. Sleep deprivation causes poor attention on tasks requiring vigilance. Relevant examples of usually routine activities that require much vigilance are administration of anesthetics and being alert to an important clue in the midst of a loquacious interview. Sleep deprivation also causes dysphoric mood. Practically no one would dispute that attentiveness and a positive attitude are indispensable for good patient care. Hence, both for

Physicians often minimize patient complaints about sleep and fatigue because:

- Their training as students and residents forced them to ignore their own sleep needs, often by working all night and being sleepy all day.
- They continue to be sleep-deprived themselves, as is much of society.
- Most physicians had no formal exposure to sleep medicine in training.
- The field of sleep medicine is still establishing itself, often with various levels of enthusiasm and disdain from both established fields of medicine and health care administrators.

Table 1
Consequences of Sleep Deprivation for Physicians in Training

Group	Number	Result	Source
Interns	14	EKG interpretation errors up 84% and attitude poor when sleep deprived	*N Engl J Med* 1970; 285: 201–203
Surgery residents	33 video tapes of surgery	Inferior performance by residents with less sleep compared to control residents	*J Surg Res* 1972; 12: 83–86
Anesthesia residents	21	Decreased performance on anesthesiology task after being on call	*J Clin Monit* 1987; 3: 22–24
Pediatrics residents	45	Slower umbilical artery catheterization time when fatigued, but other measures unchanged	*Acad Med* 1989; 64: 29–32
Second-year emergency room residents	10	Less thorough patient evaluations when fatigued	*NY State J Med* 1988; 88: 10–14

future diagnosis of sleep disorders and for future care of patients, physicians-in-training themselves need better sleep.

Thus, inadequately trained about sleep disorders, inured to sleep deprivation during their formative years, and often still getting insufficient sleep when in practice, physicians simply fail to appreciate how frequently sleepy patients appear at the office. Until physician training itself is changed, physicians will not recognize that sleepy patients are sick, have frequent accidents, and have a lower quality of life.

Sleep medicine might enhance a managed care system because:

- The treatment of sleep apnea and insomnia should help prevent cardiovascular and psychiatric illness, thereby making their detection and treatment cost-effective.
- The treatment of sleep disorders improves quality of life and should improve patient satisfaction.

---

3. SLEEP MEDICINE AND MANAGED CARE

Recognition and effective treatment of sleep disorders are especially relevant for managed care organizations. Managed care initiatives have caused considerable uproar among sleep medicine specialists, many of whom perceive a threat to their livelihoods. The specialists fear that sleep medicine will become a casualty of ruthless MBAs in search of profits. In contrast, primary care physicians in prepaid health plans might be getting the attention they deserve and feel confident. In the longer term, however, managed health plans will require both primary care physicians who are well informed about sleep disorders and sleep medicine specialists. Sleep medicine is an essential part of any well-managed health plan for several reasons.

3.1. Sleep Medicine as Preventive Medicine

The first reason that sleep medicine is relevant to managed care is something that the specialists have overlooked: sleep medicine is often preventive medicine. Patients with sleep disorders present golden opportunities for prevention of other serious diseases, in addition to treatment of the sleep disorders themselves. Figure 2 shows the increased risk of diabetes, OSA, hypertension, and cardiac mortality with increasing body weight. Many patients who have severe sleep apnea have a body mass index (BMI)—a measure of weight corrected for height expressed as kilograms divided by the square of the height in meters— of 32 or more. At that BMI, nearly 20% of patients may have diabetes, and a significant number will turn out to have elevated cholesterol, hypertension, or knee joint pain, all of which can be helped by weight loss or more specific therapies. If such patients experience a good result from continuous positive airway pressure (CPAP) therapy, their increased energy and renewed cooperation can often be translated into successful treatment of previously unrecognized or intractable risk factors. Thus, taking care of a sleep complaint opens the door for other health-promoting measures.

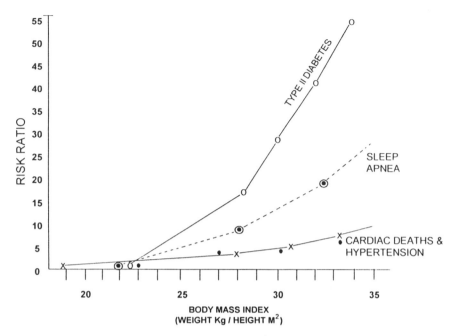

Fig. 2. Risks due to obesity. Data about type II diabetes, hypertension, and cardiac deaths adapted from the article by W. W. Gibbs, which is cited in the suggested readings section at the end of this chapter. The data on sleep apnea were adapted from Young, T., Palta, M., Dempsey, J., and colleagues. (1993) The occurrence of sleep-disordered breathing among middle-aged adults. *N Engl J Med* 328: 1230–1235.

3.2. Diagnosis and Treatment of Sleep Disorders Is Cost-Effective

Current evidence indicates that treatment of sleep disorders prevents psychiatric morbidity, heart disease, stroke, and accidents. A longitudinal study by Ford and Kamerow has linked disturbed sleep to psychiatric disease. Over a six month period, patients with chronic insomnia and insomnia of recent onset had a 35-fold greater risk of depression than persons who had no insomnia or whose insomnia was resolved. Whether insomnia is an early symptom of developing depression, insomnia is the actual cause of the depression, or some combination of both will require additional research. Whatever the cause and effect relationship of insomnia to depression, prompt recognition and vigorous treatment of insomnia should reduce depression's substantial morbidity. Because of links between insomnia, anxiety, and substance abuse, recognition and treatment of insomnia may reduce the impacts of those disorders as well.

There is strong epidemiological evidence that OSA is associated with hypertension, heart disease, stroke, and accidents of all types. Treatment of OSA with tracheostomy reduces mortality, and it is likely that CPAP can achieve a similar reduction in deaths and complications.

A recent analysis for a prepaid health plan reveals that the benefits of diagnosis and treatment of insomnia and OSA, the two most prevalent sleep disorders, outweigh the costs of maintaining a sleep disorders center. At Scripps Clinic, Steven Poceta, Merrill Mitler, Milton Erman, and this author estimated that treatment of sleep apnea could save a 100,000 member capitated health plan more than $500,000 per year by preventing myocardial infarction, stroke, hypertension, and accidents. The potential savings from treatment of insomnia for a plan of this size were about $275,000. The total savings from prevention of complications from OSA and insomnia more than offset the costs of diagnosis and treatment of sleep disorders, which were estimated to be $690,000 (about $0.58 per member per month for the prepaid health care plan). However, economic estimates such as these must be taken with a grain of salt. To realize the savings to the plan and the benefits for the patients, cooperative interaction of primary care physicians and sleep specialists would be essential.

Future prospective studies will more firmly quantify the linkages of sleep disorders to morbidity and mortality. A list of some ongoing longitudinal sleep research studies in the United States and Canada is found in Table 2. These investigations will provide direct evidence about which treatments work and how well they work. But for the moment, indirect evidence favors treatment of sleep disorders to prevent heart disease, stroke, accidents, and major depression.

3.3. Patient Satisfaction

A growing number of patients are well aware of the impacts of poor sleep on their health and performance. Proper treatment of sleep disorders enhances the patient's satisfaction with the whole range of medical care received. Increased patient well-being reflects favorably on the primary care physician, the consultant, and the health plan. Properly applied, sleep medicine can be an excellent marketing initiative for a health plan and a way for physicians to build up a cadre of loyal and healthy patients.

4. QUALITY OF LIFE AND ITS MEASUREMENT

A patient with frequent sleep disruption lives as if surrounded by fog; the world never appears clear or crisp. Pleasures are blunted. Important events are overlooked or missed entirely because of daytime sleepiness.

Table 2
Longitudinal Studies of Sleep Disorders Currently in Progress

Name	Principal investigator	Subject	Anticipated completion date
Wisconsin Sleep Cohort Study	T Young, PhD, University of Wisconsin	Morbidity and mortality of OSA	1998
Sleep and Mental Disorders Study	D. Ford, MD, Johns Hopkins University	Effect of treatment of insomnia on psychiatric outcomes	1996
Canadian CPAP and Dental Appliance Trial	A. Lowe, DDS, University of British Columbia	Comparison of CPAP and dental appliance treatment for OSA	1999
Sleep Heart Health Study	NHLBI and six universities	OSA contribution to heart disease and stroke risk	1999
Pharyngoplasty Cooperative Study	G. Sloan, University of North Carolina	Multi-center trial of pharyngoplasty	1998

Insomniacs believe that their lives are blunted by poor quality sleep, even though their actual daytime sleepiness is less than that of normal subjects (Fig. 2). Hence, besides the risks of accidents and complicating diseases, people with sleep complaints perceive a significant reduction in quality of life.

How can a person's perceptions and experiences, as tempered by beliefs and expectations, be captured as a measurable quantity? Many of the components of quality of life cannot be observed directly but can be approximated by the person's responses to a set of carefully designed questions. Sensitive and reliable questionnaires that address each of these domains—physical functioning, psychological adjustment, and work performance—do exist. Responses to such questionnaires can be used in studies of therapy to adjust simple survival according to its quality, so-called quality-adjusted life years (QALYs). The validity of such methods remains under some debate, because individual circumstances and philosophical outlook alter—and at times overshadow—the ravages of disease; there is also a range of individual reactions. Nonetheless, the important advance in medical practice is taking quality of life into account during outcome measurements.

4.1. Quality of Life for Sleep Apnea Patients

Recently, a group of Canadian researchers determined how patients with sleep apnea rated their lives before and after CPAP treatment. The substantial symptomatic improvements in daytime sleepiness, mood, and concentration after treatment translated into a median gain of 5.4 full QALYs for each treated individual. The cost of treatment per patient (as distinguished from the price) is difficult to determine, but is unlikely to exceed $1000 per patient per year, which is inexpensive when compared to other established medical interventions.

5. THE IMPACT OF TECHNOLOGY

If untreated, sleep disorders erode the quality of patients' lives. Effective therapy for sleep disturbances is available. However, sleep disorders are so common that even the combined efforts of primary care physicians and sleep specialists will not reach all patients who currently need help. Somehow, physicians' efforts must be extended and augmented.

The current diagnostic standard for sleep disorders is polysomnography (PSG). PSG cvolved as a clinical research method, with little regard for widespread practical application. PSG is inconvenient, cumbersome, labor-intensive, and expensive. Even after 30 years of use as a research tool, important questions about the reliability and validity of PSG remain unanswered.

Reassessment of clinical indications for PSG is currently underway, because of increased demand for cost-effective diagnosis. One initiative, a review of the indications for PSG and other sleep tests by a taskforce of the American Sleep Disorders Association (ASDA), was accomplished during 1996 and published in 1997. Conclusions were based on evidence from studies published in peer-reviewed journals. For the most part, the ASDA recommendations resemble the diagnostic approaches described by authors of the preceding chapters of this book.

As valuable as the newly published ASDA practice parameters may be, they will be superceded as rapidly as they appear in print. Well-designed clinical investigations always lag behind technical innovations and financial forces. For that reason, the remainder of this section on technology extrapolates beyond the ASDA report and other published practice parameters. New technology and creative protocols will prove crucial for expansion of diagnosis and therapy of sleep disorders.

5.1. Portable Sleep Tests

Too few sleep centers equipped with traditional polygraphs are available to meet real needs. Building more sleep centers may not be the best use of additional health care dollars, either to improve patients' sleep or to improve overall health. Portable sleep studies hold out considerable promise, because sleep at home may be more typical than what occurs at a sleep center, in addition to being less costly.

The reliability and validity of unattended portable sleep studies is the subject of ongoing debate. Standard PSG undoubtedly makes valid quantitative measurements of physiological variables. However, both standard PSG and portable sleep studies must surmount two obstacles: biological variability of sleep and sleep disorders limit the utility of a single night recording, and the most relevant physiological variables are not measured directly.

Biological variability is most evident for insomnia, which is also the most widespread sleep complaint. Actigraphy or the combination of actigraphy with a light monitor, made possible by recent development of miniaturized wrist recorders, allows estimation of activity and sleep in one-minute increments for a whole week. Numerous studies have shown that actigraphic measurements have a 70–90% correlation with sleep/wake status, as assessed by PSG.

Light exposure and activity under natural conditions during two successive 24-hour periods for a patient discussed later in this chapter are shown in Fig. 3. The variation of activity and estimated sleep between the two days is evident. The results of activity monitoring often differ sharply from the patient estimates of sleep time. In patients who claim "no sleep at all," but whose light/activity recordings demonstrate estimated sleep time per day of six to eight hours (including naps), sleep restriction therapy can be particularly effective treatment. Pharmacological approaches can be reserved for patients in whom sleep restriction fails. Prolonged recordings of activity are crucial for the estimation of circadian rhythm disturbances, especially sleep disorders in shift workers; for such disturbances, actigraphy is an invaluable diagnostic tool.

Biological variability night to night occurs in patients with sleep apnea and periodic limb movements of sleep (PLMS). For diagnosis of possible sleep apnea, actigraphy improves the validity of unattended portable respiratory studies, especially those that do not include a measure of sleep. When there is no reliable estimate of actual sleep time, the total recording period must be used to calculate the respiratory disturbance indices; this is inaccurate and leads to underestimation of the index. Even though actigraphic estimation of sleep is imperfect, the respiratory disturbance indices calculated using actigraphic sleep estimates are very close to those obtained with electroencephalographic (EEG) determination of sleep.

When portable sleep studies for detecting sleep-related breathing problems include body position and snoring microphone, as well as actigraphic sleep estimation, the accuracy of results approximates those from standard PSG. If electrodes malfunction, if the patient has difficulty sleeping, or if a false negative study is suspected on clinical

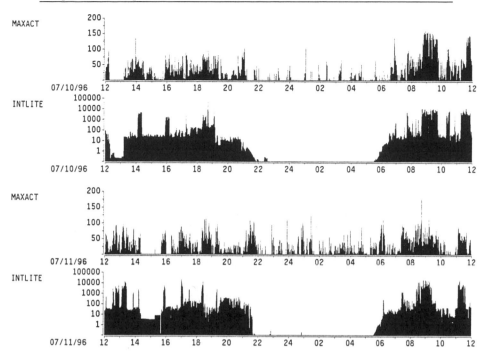

Fig. 3. Graphic display of two days of light and activity monitoring. Four rows of data are displayed. The first, MAXACT, is the maximum activity for each one minute recording epoch starting at noon on 7/10/96 and concluding at noon the following day. The first day's activity data continue into the second 24 hour recording period, which is displayed in the third row. The second and fourth rows show light intensity (INTLITE) on a logarithmic scale. The light readings are simultaneous with the activity data in the row just above. Note that daytime and nighttime activity levels vary considerably between the two periods shown, but light exposure appears to be more uniform for this patient.

grounds, the portable sleep study can be repeated. Hence, actigraphy is an innovation that deals with the problems of inadequate sampling and biological variability of sleep disorders and improves the validity of portable sleep studies.

A second obstacle for sleep studies of all types is explicit measurement of the physiological variable of interest. For example, the belts around the chest and abdomen used to measure respiratory effort may give false-negative readings during the course of the night. Rhythmic airflow may continue in an obese subject, even when chest and abdominal movements are difficult to detect. Esophageal pressures may indicate increased upper airway resistance associated with fragmented sleep, even when chest and abdominal movements and airflow appear normal.

Insensitive indirect measurements explain why the upper airway resistance syndrome (UARS) can be missed on PSG or why a patient with mostly "central apneas" on PSG may respond to CPAP therapy. New portable studies that estimate upper airway resistance using sensitive nasal flow sensors might overcome some of the shortcomings of indirect measurements. Coupled with body position determination and actigraphic estimation of sleep, portable devices that measure upper airway resistance might provide direct cost-effective diagnosis of sleep-related breathing disorders, including UARS.

5.2. Digital EEG

Lacking a comprehensive theory to define the essential components of good sleep, sleep quality must be measured indirectly. EEG determination of sleep architecture and fragmentation is the best objective yardstick of good sleep. At this time, there is no substitute for EEG in the assessment of sleep quality and for titration of CPAP therapy for sleep-related breathing problems, although its clinical utility is not universally proven or accepted. Nonetheless, accepting the necessity for EEG measurement, digital recording of EEG opens the door for more precise, sensitive, and cost-effective analysis of EEG. Digitized EEG can be analyzed by computer, automatically aligned with other physiological measurements during sleep, and presented in a compressed display. The computer analysis and data reduction lessen the time required for sleep staging, and the staging is more uniform. Interpretation is easier, because the real strength of correlations among the physiological variables can be seen at once, as shown in Fig. 4. Details can be checked by sampling relevant portions of the raw data. An additional benefit has to do with storage of the records: magnetic disks require less space and are more accessible than paper records and eliminate costly problems with archiving.

5.3. Automatic CPAP Titration

Unattended CPAP titration using a computer-regulated device is feasible, but its benefits are not yet clear, and the results compared to in-laboratory titration are preliminary. Savings in labor costs might be substantial when titration is automated, and titration can be done very quickly when pressure changes are based on the upper airway resistance. The final pressure may be more physiological than that determined by the technician's observations of hypopneas, snoring, and paradoxical respiration in various body positions and sleep stages. Nevertheless, getting a comfortable fit for the CPAP mask at an optimum pressure; reassuring the anxious, first-time patient; and encourag-

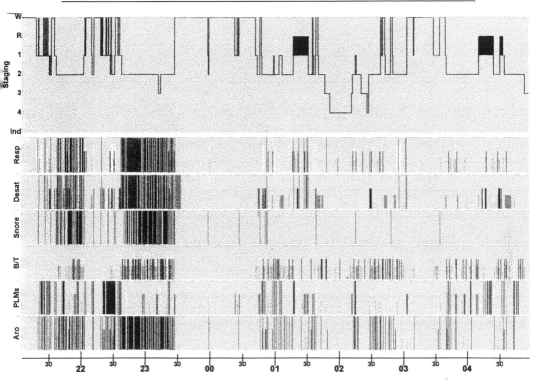

Fig. 4. Graphic summary of a polysomnogram recorded on a digital polygraph. From bottom to top, the eight rows in this graphic are 1. the time line of the recording, 2. the number of EEG arousals, 3. periodic limb movements (PLM), 4. bradycardias and tachycardias, 5. snoring, 6. oxygen desaturations, 7. apneas and hypopneas, and 8. sleep staging. Note the strong temporal correlations among apneas and hypopneas, snoring, oxygen desaturations, and EEG arousals. CPAP therapy, started about 2330, reduced apneas and hypopneas, desaturations, and snoring for the remainder of the test period. PLMs do occur through the test period, but correlate less well with arousals than do the respiratory disturbances.

ing the patient to give the apparatus a good trial all require human skills: they are not necessarily automatable. Perhaps titration that is both automated and attended will result in the best long-term compliance with CPAP therapy.

Besides new technologies such as automated CPAP, new clinical strategies and protocols will also be developed to improve the diagnosis and treatment of patients with sleep disorders. As mentioned above, it is not feasible currently for all of the patients estimated to have sleep apnea to go through two nights of sleep laboratory testing. Protocols that adequately screen patients for sleep disorders—both by clinical assessment and by initial testing—must be combined with efficient treatment protocols. For example, a pilot study at Scripps Clinic is being performed in which patients suspected sleep apnea are screened with overnight oximetry (with recording and computer analysis). If certain clinical and oximetry criteria are met, the patients are prescribed CPAP set at a pressure determined by a protocol that takes into account severity of apnea, initial response, and comfort of the patient to the CPAP and is adjusted based on the first several nights of treatment. This trial seems to indicate that, in some patients, diagnosis and treatment is so straightforward (given proper physician knowledge and experience), that in-laboratory studies can be avoided entirely.

5.4. Drug Design

Technology will improve therapy at least as much as it improves diagnosis. New medications will be key weapons with which primary care physicians and sleep medicine specialists combat insomnia, restless legs syndrome, PLMS disorder, and the obesity that precipitates sleep apnea.

5.4.1. ANTIDEPRESSANTS AND HYPNOTICS

Disturbed sleep—especially early morning awakening—is strongly associated with major depression. The success of antidepressant therapy for this specific kind of insomnia opens avenues of considerable promise for future drug development. Serotonin metabolism and the myriad of serotonin receptor subtypes appear to play an important role in sleep and depression, so more selective agents to modulate sleep may be designed by attention to specific serotonin receptor subtypes. That such drugs could improve the subjective quality of sleep for insomniacs without depression appears quite possible. If so, a biochemical classification and more rational treatment for insomnia could develop. Biotechnological design of agents to act on specific receptor subtypes may prove very important for treatment and understanding of PLMS and the restless legs syndrome, as well.

The underlying biochemistry and neuropharmacology of sleep itself is a field in which there is potential for great advances; for example, the recent discovery of a previously unknown compound, isolated from the cerebrospinal fluid (CSF) of sleep-deprived cats has been shown to induce sleep and to lower body temperature in rats. Modern chemical techniques have synthesized the compound (called oleamide), and work is proceeding on identifying its biosynthetic and metabolic pathways (*see* Cravatt, et al.).

5.4.2. OBESITY AGENTS

Recent scientific advances have opened exciting prospects for obesity treatments. Genetic research on the obese mouse has identified five

Table 3
Sleep Medicine on the Internet

Organization	Internet address
American Sleep Disorders Association	http://www.asda.org
Circadian Technologies, Inc.	http://www.circadian.com
NASA Fatigue Countermeasures Program	http://www-afo.arc.nasa.gov/zteam/
Phantom Sleep Page	http://www.newtechpub.com
Quietsleep (oral appliances)	http://www.quietsleep.com
ResMed Company	http://www.resmed.com.au
Sleep Medicine Home Page	http://www.users.cloud9.net/~thorpy
Sleep Net	http://www.sleepnet.com/
The Sleep Well	http://www-leland.stanford.edu/~dement/
(political action about sleep disorders)	
Restless legs syndrome foundation	http://www.rls.org

pivotal mutations that may be used for weight control. The gene products of two of the five mutations now are known; one is leptin—a fat cell hormone—and the other is a leptin-receptor protein, the activation of which suppresses appetite. Other research has shown that neuropeptide Y stimulates and cholecystokinin suppresses appetite in humans. Pharmacological agents to promote or block each of these pathways are under development.

5.5. Information Technology

How can primary care physicians best obtain information about diagnosis, prognosis, and treatment of their patients who have sleep disorders? One method is consultation; referral of a patient to a sleep specialist often yields insights about current methods of diagnosis and treatment. However, consultation is not always feasible. Fortunately, the interested physician can supplement his or her knowledge by use of information from the National Library of Medicine's (NLM) vast Medline database. Other relevant information can be obtained through the Internet; several Internet addresses are shown in Table 3.

6. DIFFICULT SLEEP PROBLEMS

With a grasp of the sleep disorders reviewed in the nine previous chapters of this book, management of many patients' sleep problems will be straightforward. Nevertheless, clinical situations that appear direct may really contain pitfalls; the pathways that need navigation can rapidly exceed any physician's capacity for informal estimation. Rigorous methods, such as decision analysis, may be required to solve complex problems.

6.1. Sleep Medicine Consultation

For patients who have difficult sleep problems, a sleep medicine consultation is an efficient first step. Sleep medicine consultation provides several advantages: a directed interview by the specialist; intimate knowledge of diagnostic and therapeutic technology; practical experience with results of interventions; and experience with the pitfalls of sleep disorders. Of the advantages, the experience with interviewing and knowledge of usual outcomes is most valuable and can only be gained through constant practice. In contrast, the primary physician's strength resides in a more complete knowledge of the patient and the patient's environment, information not easily obtained by a consultant. A discussion between the primary physician and the consultant combines their insights, leading to the most effective use of diagnostic tests and treatments. Either physician acting alone may not have the groundwork for optimum decision-making.

6.2. Decision Analysis for Complex Sleep Medicine Problems

Nevertheless, medical decisions sometimes exceed the information processing capability of any primary care or specialist physician at bedside. Most often, things become too complicated when diagnosis and treatment involve considerable risks and costs as well as distinct benefits. Consider what at first appears to be a simple example: should an unattended portable sleep study rather than a standard PSG be used to diagnose a patient with suspected sleep apnea?

The patient has a high probability of OSA. He snores loudly and continually when asleep, which keeps his wife awake. She has noted apneas. The patient's body mass index is 31 Kg/M^2, and he is hypertensive. His ESS score is 12. From this history, the probability of OSA is at least 70%.

Figure 5 is a decision tree that shows the probabilities and costs of the various diagnostic and therapeutic tests. The only choice in this decision tree is the first branch point—whether to start with a portable study or a sleep center PSG. There are seven possible outcomes, which are from the top:

1. Severe OSA found by the portable study and followed by a CPAP titration.
2. Milder OSA for which a dental appliance is appropriate.
3. No OSA (and no final diagnosis for the patient's complaints).
4. Severe OSA that is not evident until too late in the night for a split-night study with CPAP titration.
5. Severe OSA with CPAP titration in one night.
6. Milder OSA for which a dental appliance is useful.
7. Another sleep disorder diagnosed by PSG.

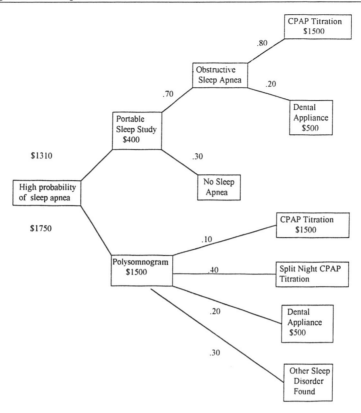

Fig. 5. A decision tree showing the outcomes of sleep diagnostic tests. Note that, in this particular example, the outcomes from the choices listed in the two major branches are asymmetrical. The 30% of patients given a portable sleep study who receive no definitive final diagnosis are discussed in the text.

The decision tree is asymmetrical, because the information provided by the portable study in not as complete as what is provided by the standard PSG.

Folding back the decision tree to determine the costs of the two pathways—portable sleep study versus standard PSG—involves multiplying the probability of each outcome by its cost and adding up the results at each branch. In this example, the portable study appears to be the most cost-effective way to proceed ($1350 vs. $1750). However, what will be done for the patient with outcome number 3, who has no sleep apnea? If a definite diagnosis is required, a standard PSG may be needed. If outcome of standard PSG is added to branch number 3, the cost for the portable pathway rises to $1760, which is actually more expensive than ordering the standard PSG in the first place!

In other instances, the costs and probabilities will be different, but the circumstances may be even more complicated. For example, a complete decision analysis on a different sleep patient (not shown) had 64 possible outcomes. That analysis revealed that an initial standard PSG would be the most cost-effective diagnostic strategy. For the reader who wants to become more skillful with clinical decision making, including decision analysis, Sackett and colleagues' book, *Clinical Epidemiology*, is an excellent place to start.

For patients with suspected sleep-related breathing disorders whose pretest probability of OSA is less than 70%, it turns out that standard PSG is almost always a better choice than a portable study. When diagnosis is uncertain, the less costly portable test often has to be followed by a complete PSG anyway. The "bottom line" is that cost-effectiveness may not be established even in "simple" situations, unless a rigorous analysis of all possible outcomes, namely a decision tree, is used. However, the assumptions that go into the model are not always correct, or data are lacking, or the situation is different from place to place, specialist to specialist.

7. THE PRIMARY CARE PHYSICIAN'S ROLE

The primary care physician's role in the diagnosis and treatment of sleep disorders should emphasize preventive medicine rather than high technology. Among the skills required for identification of patients who may have sleep problems are; being alert to possible sleep problems in the first place; recognition of whether the patients identified are ready for treatment; education of patients about sleep and sleep disorders; arranging timely consultation for serious sleep disorders; follow-up of treatments; and health promotion.

7.1. Case Finding

Foremost among the skills required for identification of sleep disorders are: the temerity to interrogate the patient about daytime sleepiness, snoring, apneas, insomnia, and depression; a knack for listening; and the interest to solve sleep problems that are identified. The ESS helps identify excessive daytime sleepiness, but it is best to review the responses with the both the patient and spouse, if possible. The Beck Depression Inventory helps to differentiate depression-induced fatigue from true sleepiness. Sleep diaries and questions about extra sleep on weekends are essential to identify circadian disturbances and insufficient sleep syndrome.

7.2. Assessment of Readiness for Intervention

Physicians expect patients to change long-term behaviors quickly to preserve health, but patients often are not ready to take suggestions about

The primary care physician should:

- Identify the patient with a sleep disorder.
- Assess the patient's readiness for change and intervention.
- Begin patient education and initial treatment regimens.
- Refer appropriate patients to sleep medicine specialists.

Table 4
Process of Change:
Stages for Behavior Intervention

Stage	Clues	Intervention
Precontemplation	Family pressure, but denies any interest in the subject	Leave door open, but do not push
Contemplation	Some openness on the part of the patient	Talk about the pros and cons of taking action
Preparation	Focusing in on making a commitment	Information about a plan of action
Action	Following a course of action	Encouragement and practical advice about how to succeed
Maintenance	Goal reached	Tips about how to stay vigilant and prevent relapse

preventive medicine. Assessing readiness to change is important for long-term treatment success for CPAP treatment of OSA, sleep restriction for insomnia, smoking cessation, weight reduction, control of hypertension, lipid control by diet and medication, and many other therapies.

Prochaska and colleagues have described a "Process of Change Model" of behavior modification that helps the practicing physician know how much to intercede. The Process of Change Model includes five stages: precontemplation, contemplation, preparation, action, and maintenance. The important ideas are summarized in Table 4. Recognition of how ready the patient is for change can focus the physician's efforts, reduce frustration, and increase chances of treatment success.

7.3. Patient Education

Many sleep disorders can be diagnosed with a simple interview and treated on the spot, but it is rare that the best initial therapy is a sleeping pill. Insufficient sleep, for example, is rampant among students, people in their twenties, and achievement-centered individuals. Like other patients with excessive daytime sleepiness, patients with insufficient sleep usually have elevated scores on the ESS. Conversely, insomniacs usually have low ESS scores, and may actually be resting more than their biological requirement. Initial treatment for both groups is instruction about how much sleep is appropriate. Most sleep textbooks, including this one, contain lists of sleep hygiene measures, for example restricting bedroom activities to sex and sleep, avoiding stimulants such as caffeine in the evening, establishing a regular bedtime, and so forth. Such simple advice can be curative for many sleep problems that the primary physician will encounter.

CASE STUDY

Sorting out a patient's sleep complaints may be difficult, even for an experienced sleep medicine specialist. Consider this seventy-year-old man who described insomnia ("Most nights, I don't sleep much at all"), restless legs, and painful joints that disturbed his sleep. Tramadol, prescribed by a rheumatologist, allowed better quality sleep on some nights. He had been told that he snored loudly, but he slept alone; there were no witnessed apneas. His ESS score was 5. Body mass index was ideal: 24 kg/m^2. Facial structure and palate appeared normal.

The initial interview suggested some combination of psychophysiological insomnia, restless leg syndrome, sleep disruption by arthritis, and sleep-related respiratory disorder. Considering the variability of the manifestations, a protracted sample of this patient's sleep pattern seemed necessary, but specific testing for sleep-breathing abnormalities was needed, too. Keeping costs under control was a priority.

An unattended portable sleep study on one night revealed a respiratory disturbance index of 24 per hour, mostly groups of relatively short central hypopneas with no desaturations below 86%. The hypopneas did not correlate with the frequent limb movements, which were also present, that reduced sleep efficiency to 90% as estimated by actigraphy.

Seven days of light-activity monitoring with simultaneous sleep diary and computerized estimation of sleep revealed naps of 45–90 minutes on five days. For three of the seven nights, limb activity pattern appeared normal and the patient rated his sleep as very good. On two of the good nights, he had taken 100 mg of tramadol before retiring. The other four nights, when he did not sleep much at all by his estimation, there were very frequent limb movements; the afternoon naps did not correlate with poor quality sleep the following night. During his worst night, he took tramadol without success. Nonetheless, he appeared to average over nine hours of sleep per day, as estimated by the computer analysis of his movements.

Initial therapy with sleep restriction was not successful. Pergolide did not provide relief, judging from the sleep diary. There was no evidence of depression by the Beck Depression Inventory. A trial of cyclobenzaprine for suspected fibromyalgia did not help. The initial treatment failures led to further discussion and trials of medications. Low-dose amitriptyline and tramadol together finally resulted in a patient who was much more satisfied with both the quality of his sleep and his daytime energy.

Discussion

Decisions about the most useful sleep tests to employ, interpretation of the results of the testing, and assessment of the efficacy of interventions in this case was complicated. Sleep medicine consultation helped the primary care physician with the differential diagnosis and choice of diagnostic tests. But the family physician was best able to assess the patient's responses to therapy, and ultimately to treat the patient successfully. Although the testing helped guide initial therapy and ruled out certain conditions, the therapeutic agents were chosen on the basis of clinical judgement.

7.4. Follow-Up of Therapy

After sleep medicine consultation and sleep testing have been completed, follow-up of the patient is necessary to ensure a good outcome. Listen to the patient, but interview the bedpartner as well, in order to gain crucial insight into changes in daytime function, nocturnal events, and compliance with therapy. Newer CPAP machines contain computer chips that monitor actual usage at pressure, which allows the physician to improve poor compliance or prescribe alternative therapy. The ESS can document response to treatment in patients with initial daytime sleepiness. Sleep diaries are useful to document response to treatment for insomnia and periodic limb movement disorder.

7.5. Health Promotion

Specialist physicians spend most of their efforts on patients' diseases. In contrast, primary care physicians deliver a wide range of preventive care services. Preventive care includes: health enhancement, usually counseling about nutrition, physical activity, and adjustment to life stages; risk avoidance, for example, immunizations, seat belt use, bicycle helmets; risk reduction, e.g., cholesterol control to prevent heart disease; early identification of diseases; and complication reduction, for example reducing heart failure by treatment of OSA.

When treating patients with sleep disorders, the major preventive medicine opportunity lies in risk reduction, early identification, and complication reduction. Of particular relevance are treatment of obesity in OSA patients and treatment of depression and drug habituation in patients with insomnia. Seize the opportunity provided by increased wakefulness in treated sleep apnea patients to encourage diet and exercise. As fatigue or depression lifts and sleep improves, encourage the patient to cope with underlying sources of stress and unhappiness, and help patients avoid sedatives, alcohol, and nonprescription sleep aids.

8. THE BEGINNING

You have indeed finished this book, but your job with the patients in your waiting room is just beginning. You now have the tools to improve their sleep, make some headway against risk factors, and so improve their long-term health. Treating patients with sleep disorders is fun, and the results can bring a smile to your own face even at the end of a long, tiring day at the office.

SUGGESTED READINGS

1. Indications for Polysomnography Task Force, American Sleep Disorders Association Standards of Practice Committee. Practice parameters for polysomnography and related procedures. *Sleep* 1997; 20: 406–422.
2. Ford DE, Kamerow DB. Epidemiologic study of sleep disturbance and psychiatric disorders: an opportunity for prevention? *JAMA* 1989; 262: 1479–1484.
3. Gibbs WW. Gaining on fat. *Scientific American*. 1996; 275: 88–94.
4. Johns MW. Sleepiness in different situations measured by the Epworth Sleepiness Scale. *Sleep* 1994; 17: 703–710.
5. Johnson SF, Erman MK, Poceta JS, Mitler MM. Sleep disorders, preventive medicine, and prepaid health care, in Pascualy R. (Director) *Managed Care Strategies for Sleep Medicine.* Association of Professional Sleep Societies, Rochester, MN, 1996, pp. 1–31.
6. Prochaska JO, Velicer WF, Rossi JS, et al. Stages of change and decisional balance for 12 problem behaviors. *Health Psychology* 1994; 13: 39–46.
7. Sackett DL, Haynes RB, Guyatt GH, Tugwell P. Clinical Epidemiology, 2nd ed. Little Brown, Boston, 1991.
8. Testa MA, Simonson DC. Current concepts: assessment of quality-of-life outcomes. *N Engl J Med* 1996; 334: 841–848.
9. Tousignant P, Cosio MG, Levy RD, Groome PA. Quality adjusted life years added by treatment of obstructive sleep apnea. *Sleep* 1994; 17: 52–60.
10. Cravatt BF, Prospero-Garcia O, Siuzdak G, Gilula NB, Henriksen SJ, Boger DL, Lerner RA. Chemical characterization of a family of brain lipids that induce sleep. *Science* 1995; 268: 1506–1509.

APPENDIX

This table is taken from the International Classification of Sleep Disorders (ICSD), published by the American Sleep Disorders Association in 1997. It can serve as an overview of how sleep disorders are organized and classified by experts, and will help the reader conceptualize some of the conditions discussed in this book. Not all conditions listed are discussed in the text; however, many of the names are self-evident, and for more information, the reader should consult the ICSD.

	ICD-9-CM code recommendation
1. Dyssomnias	
A. Intrinsic Sleep Disorders	
1. Psychophysiologic insomnia	307.42
2. Sleep state misperception	307.49
3. Idiopathic insomnia	780.52
4. Narcolepsy	347
5. Recurrent hypersomnia	780.54
6. Idiopathic hypersomnia	780.54
7. Posttraumatic hypersomnia	780.54
8. Obstructive sleep apnea syndrome	780.53
9. Central sleep apnea syndrome	780.51
10. Central alveolar hypoventilation syndrome	780.51
11. Periodic limb movement disorder	780.52
12. Restless legs syndrome	780.52
13. Intrinsic sleep disorder not otherwise specified	780.52
B. Extrinsic sleep disorders	
1. Inadequate sleep hygiene	307.41
2. Environmental sleep disorder	780.52
3. Altitude insomnia	289.0
4. Adjustment sleep disorder	307.41
5. Insufficient sleep syndrome	307.49
6. Limit-setting sleep disorder	307.42
7. Sleep-onset association disorder	307.42
8. Food allergy insomnia	780.52
9. Nocturnal eating syndrome	780.52
10. Hypnotic-dependent sleep disorder	780.52
11. Stimulant-dependent sleep disorder	780.52
12. Alcohol-dependent sleep disorder	780.52
13. Toxin-Induced sleep disorder	780.54
14. Extrinsic sleep disorder not otherwise specified	780.52
C. Circadian rhythm sleep disorders	
1. Time zone change (jet lag) syndrome	307.45
2. Shift work sleep disorder	307.45
3. Irregular sleep-wake pattern	307.45
4. Delayed sleep-phase syndrome	780.55
5. Advanced sleep-phase syndrome	780.55
6. Non-24-hour sleep-wake disorder	780.55
7. Circadian rhythm sleep disorder not otherwise specified	780.55

	ICD-9-CM code recommendation
2. Parasomnias	
A. Arousal disorders	
1. Confusional arousals	307.46
2. Sleep walking	307.46
3. Sleep terrors	307.46
B. Sleep-wake transition disorders	
1. Rhythmic movement disorder	307.3
2. Sleep starts	307.47
3. Sleep talking	307.47
4. Nocturnal leg cramps	729.82
C. Parasomnias usually associated with REM sleep	
1. Nightmares	307.47
2. Sleep paralysis	780.56
3. Impaired sleep-related penile erections	780.56
4. Sleep-related painful erections	780.56
5. REM sleep-related sinus arrest	780.56
6. REM sleep behavior disorder	780.59
D. Other parasomnias	
1. Sleep bruxism	306.8
2. Sleep enuresis	780.56
3. Sleep-related abnormal swallowing syndrome	780.56
4. Nocturnal paroxysmal dystonia	780.59
5. Sudden unexplained nocturnal death syndrome	780.59
6. Primary snoring	780.53
7. Infant sleep apnea	770.80
8. Congenital central hypoventilation syndrome	770.81
9. Sudden infant death syndrome	798.0
10. Benign neonatal sleep myoclonus	780.9
11. Other parasomnia not otherwise specified	780.59
3. Medical/psychiatric sleep disorders	
A. Associated with mental disorders	
1. Psychoses	292–319
2. Mood disorders	292–299
3. Anxiety disorders	300
4. Panic disorder	300
5. Alcoholism	303
B. Associated with neurological disorders	
1. Cerebral degenerative disorders	330–337
2. Dementia	331
3. Parkinsonism	332–333
4. Fatal familial insomnia	337.9
5. Sleep-related epilepsy	345
6. Electrical status epilepticus of sleep	345.8
7. Sleep-related headaches	346

	ICD-9-CM code
C. Associated with other medical disorders	recommendation
1. Sleeping sickness	086
2. Nocturnal cardiac ischemia	411–414
3. Chronic obstructive pulmonary disease	490–494
4. Sleep-related asthma	493
5. Sleep-related gastroesophageal reflux	530.1
6. Peptic ulcer disease	531–534
7. Fibromyalgia syndrome	729.1

4. Proposed sleep disorders	
1. Short sleeper	307.49
2. Long sleeper	307.49
3. Subwakefulness syndrome	307.47
4. Fragmentary myoclonus	780.59
5. Sleep hyperhidrosis	780.8
6. Menstrual-associated sleep disorder	780.54
7. Pregnancy-associated sleep disorder	780.59
8. Terrifying hypnagogic hallucinations	307.47
9. Sleep-related neurogenic tachypnea	780.53
10. Sleep-related laryngospasm	780.59
11. Sleep choking syndrome	307.42

APPENDIX 2

Manufacturers of bright light boxes

Apollo Light Systems
352 West 1060 South
Orem, UT 84058
Phone: 800-545-9667

Enviro-Med
1600 SE 141st Ave.
Vancouver, WA 98684
Phone: 800-222-DAWN

Sun Box
19217 Orbit Drive
Gaithersburg, MD 20879
Phone: 800-548-3968

Northern Light Technologies
8971 Henri Bourassa West
Montreal, Canada H4S 1P7
Phone: 800-263-0066

Manufacturers of nasal CPAP machines

Respironics Inc.
1501 Ardmore Blvd.
Pittsburgh, PA 15221
Phone: 800-345-6443

Healthdyne Technologies
1255 Kennestone Circle
Marietta, GA 30066
Phone: 800-421-8754 or 770-499-1212

ResMed Corp.
10121 Carol Canyon Rd.
San Diego, CA 92131
Phone: 800-424-0737 or 619-689-2400

Nellcor Puritan Bennett
4280 Hacienda Dr.
Pleasanton, CA 94588
Phone: 800-635-5267 or 510-463-4000

INDEX